D0915037

The Past, Present and Future of Home Health Care

Guest Editor

PETER A. BOLING, MD

CLINICS IN GERIATRIC MEDICINE

www.geriatric.theclinics.com

February 2009 • Volume 25 • Number 1

SAUNDERS an imprint of ELSEVIER, Inc.

W.B. SAUNDERS COMPANY

A Division of Elsevier Inc.

1600 John F. Kennedy Blvd., Suite 1800. Philadelphia, Pennsylvania 19103-2899

http://www.theclinics.com

CLINICS IN GERIATRIC MEDICINE Volume 25, Number 1
February 2009 ISSN 0749–0690, ISBN-13: 978-1-4377-0480-8, ISBN-10: 1-4377-0480-8

Editor: Yonah Korngold

Clinics in Geriatric Medicine (ISSN 0749-0690) is published quarterly by Elsevier Inc., 360 Park Avenue South, New York, NY 10010-1710. Months of issue are February, May, August, and November. Business and Editorial Offices: 1600 John F. Kennedy Blvd., Suite 1800, Philadelphia, PA 191023-2899. Customer Service Office: 6277 Sea Harbor Drive, Orlando, FL 32887-4800. Periodicals postage paid at New York, NY, and additional mailing offices. Subscription prices is $208.00 per year (US individuals), $353.00 per year (US institutions), $271.00 per year (Canadian individuals), $440.00 per year (Canadian institutions), $288.00 per year (foreign individuals) and $440.00 per year (foreign institutions). Foreign air speed delivery is included in all *Clinics* subscription prices. All prices are subject to change without notice. POSTMASTER: Send address changes to *Clinics in Geriatric Medicine,* Elsevier Periodicals Customer Service, 6277 Sea Harbor Drive, Orlando, FL 32887-4800. **Customer Service: 1-800-654-2452 (US). From outside of the United States, call 1-314-453-7041. Fax: 1-314-453-5170. E-mail: JournalsCustomerService-usa@elsevier.com.**

Reprints. For copies of 100 or more, of articles in this publication, please contact the Commercial Reprints Department, Elsevier Inc., 360 Park Avenue South, New York, New York 10010-1710. Tel.: (212) 633-3812; Fax: (212) 462-1935, email: reprints@elsevier.com.

Clinics in Geriatric Medicine is covered in *MEDLINE/PubMed (Index Medicus), EMBASE/Excerpta Medica, Current Contents/Clinical Medicine (CC/CM),* and the *Cumulative Index to Nursing & Allied Health Literature.*

Printed in the United States of America.

Contributors

GUEST EDITOR

PETER A. BOLING, MD
Professor of Medicine, Department of Medicine, Virginia Commonwealth University, Richmond, Virginia

AUTHORS

L. ABBEY, MD
Associate Professor of General Medicine, Primary Care/Geriatrics, Virginia Commonwealth University, Richmond, Virginia

KAREN ALSTON, RN, MSN, MBA
Senior Vice President of Home Health/Chief Nurse Officer, The Visiting Nurse Association of Greater Philadelphia, Philadelphia, Pennsylvania

C. GRESHAM BAYNE, MD, FAAEM
Chairman, Janus Health, San Diego, California

JULIE LEFTWICH BEALES, MD, PhD, MSHA
Assistant Professor, Department of Internal Medicine, Virginia Commonwealth University; and Associate Chief of Staff for Geriatrics and Extended Care, VAMC, Richmond, Virginia

PETER A. BOLING, MD
Professor of Medicine, Department of Medicine, Virginia Commonwealth University, Richmond, Virginia

KENNETH BRUMMEL-SMITH, MD
Charlotte Edwards Maguire Professor and Chair, Department of Geriatrics, Florida State University College of Medicine, Tallahassee, Florida

JENNIFER CHENG, MD
Johns Hopkins Bayview Medical Center, Johns Hopkins University School of Medicine, Baltimore, Maryland

REBECCA CONANT, MD
Associate Professor, Department of Medicine, University of California, San Francisco, San Francisco, California

MARIANA DANGIOLO, MD
Assistant Professor, Department of Geriatrics, Florida State University College of Medicine, Tallahassee, Florida

LINDA DeCHERRIE, MD
Assistant Professor, Geriatrics and Adult Development and Medicine, Mount Sinai Medical Center, New York, New York

K. ERIC DeJONGE, MD
Director of Geriatrics, Section of Geriatrics and Long-Term Care, Washington Hospital Center, Washington, DC

THOMAS EDES, MD, MS
Director, Home and Community-Based Care, U.S. Department of Veterans Affairs, Washington, DC

JENNIFER HAYASHI, MD
Assistant Professor, Department of Geriatric Medicine & Gerontology, Johns Hopkins University School of Medicine, Baltimore, Maryland

HELEN KAO, MD
Assistant Professor, Department of Medicine, University of California, San Francisco, San Francisco, California

BRUCE LEFF, MD
Associate Professor, Division of Geriatric Medicine and Gerontology, Department of Medicine, Johns Hopkins University School of Medicine, Johns Hopkins Bayview Medical Center, Baltimore, Maryland

WAYNE McCORMICK, MD, MPH
Associate Professor, Department of Medicine, Division of Gerontology and Geriatric Medicine, University of Washington School of Medicine, Harborview Medical Center, Seattle, Washington

MICHAEL MONTALTO, MBBS, PhD
Director, Hospital in the Home; Epworth Hospital, Richmond Victoria; Royal Melbourne Hospital, Australia

RACHEL L. MURKOFSKY, MD, MPH
Assistant Professor of Geriatric Medicine, Department of Geriatric Medicine, John A. Burns School of Medicine, Honolulu, Hawaii

ROBERT NEWCOMER, PhD
Professor, Center for Personal Assistance Services, University of California, San Francisco, California

EDWARD RATNER, MD
Associate Professor, Department of Medicine, Division of General Medicine, University of Minnesota Medical School, Minneapolis, Minnesota

ROBERT J. ROSATI, PhD
Director of Research, Evaluation and Informatics, Center for Home Care Policy & Research, New York

THERESA SORIANO, MD, MPH
Assistant Professor, Mount Sinai School of Medicine New York, Mount Sinai Visiting Doctors Program, New York, New York

ROBYN STONE, DrPH
Executive Director, Institute for the Future of Aging Services, Washington, DC

GEORGE TALER, MD
Director of Long-Term Care, Section of Geriatrics and Long-Term Care, Washington Hospital Center, Washington, DC

Contents

> The prevalence and seriousness of elder abuse and neglect require the collaboration of health care professionals with many other disciplines for adequate assessment and intervention. The home visit provides a unique opportunity for the visitor to evaluate risk factors. Interventions and reporting depend on available resources, expertise and local reporting laws. Possible reasons for low physician and victim self-reporting are reviewed. Domestic violence persists into late life and requires diffferent approaches than dealing with caregiver burnout or self-neglect. Involvement of health professionals in educating others in the community about elder abuse and neglect may allow isolated at-risk elders to be identified.

> Assistive technologies are critical to elders maintaining independence in the home. Adequate assessment of the patient's needs, the appropriateness of the device that need, and the patient's motivation to use of a device is required for successful outcomes. A team approach is needed to ensure that devices are correctly prescribed, and the patient is taught how to use it effectively. A wide range of devices is available to support activities of daily living, mobility, home management, and safety. The use of personal computers is significantly expanding the possibility of independent living through support systems, monitoring systems, and information resources.

> Although the acute hospital is the standard venue for treating acute serious illness, it is often a difficult environment for older adults who are highly susceptible to functional decline and other iatrogenic consequences of hospital care. Hospital care is also expensive. Providing acute hospital-level care at home, in lieu of usual institutional care, is viable. As an emerging service model, the definition of hospital at home (HaH) remains unsettled. Data favor HaH models that provide substantial physician inputs and are geared toward substituting for hospital care, provide service that is highly satisfying to patients and their caregivers, are associated with less iatrogenic complications, and are less expensive. Dissemination of HaH in integrated delivery systems is feasible. Widespread dissemination of HaH in the United States will require payment reform that acknowledges the role of HaH in the health care system.

C. Gresham Bayne and Peter A. Boling

Medicare reimbursement for home visits average around $100 without ancillaries, so making 10 home visits to prevent even a single $1,000 ambulance ride is cost-neutral for Medicare. Home medical care is only an added cost if it fails to offset acute care use. The government's demographic and financial pressure suggests a need to press ahead with the enhanced mobile care model, so the explosion in point-of-care devices should continue. The main challenge is to decide which ones provide dispositive value to patients.

Jennifer Hayashi, Linda DeCherrie, Edward Ratner, and Peter A. Boling

With the rapidly aging population, it is anticipated that within two decades several million more individuals in the United States with functional impairment and serious ill health will need home health care. This article discusses workforce development, which is a critical issue for future planning, as recently highlighted by the Institute of Medicine (IOM). Key aspects of recruitment, training, and retention of home care workers are discussed, including those who provide basic support for activities of daily living as well as a variety of skilled professionals: therapists, nurses, pharmacists, and physicians. Although the geriatric workforce shortage affects all care settings, it is especially critical in home health care, in part because we are starting with far too few clinicians to meet the medical needs of homebound elderly. A combination of actions is needed, including educational programs, such as those developed by the American Academy of Home Care Physicians (AAHCP), changes in financial incentives, and changes in the culture and practice of health care, to make the home the primary focus of care for these vulnerable, underserved individuals rather than an afterthought.

Robert J. Rosati

Quality improvement is as central to home health care as to any other field of health care. With the mandated addition in 2000 of Outcome Assessment and Information Set (OASIS) and outcome-based quality improvement (OBQI), Medicare home health agencies entered a new era of documenting, tracking, and systematically improving quality. OBQI is augmented by the Medicare Quality Improvement Organization (QIO) program, which is now entering the ninth in a series of work assignments, with the tenth scope in the planning stages. Evidence has shown that applied quality improvement methods can drive better outcomes using important metrics, such as acute care hospitalization. This article reviews key findings from the past 2 decades of home care quality improvement research and public policy advances, describes specific examples of local and regional programmatic approaches to quality improvement, and forecasts near-future trends in this vital arena of home health care.

Care Transitions and Home Health Care

Peter A. Boling

Transitions of care are becoming recognized as an important area for improvement in health care quality and patient safety. Yet there remains consistent evidence from multiple studies in varied settings of failures to complete safe, effective hand-offs from one location of care to the next. Major lapses include absent or limited clinical information and care plan content, plus errors related to medications. There are identifiable problems with half or more of the transitions that occur between care settings, and adverse consequences occur in 15 to 25 percent of patients. Undoubtedly these lapses contribute to the rates of re-hospitalization in post-acute care which affect 20 to 30 percent of patients within 60 days after hospital discharge. This article reviews models of transitional care intervention that have been tested and shown to be effective including less intensive coaching or guided care approaches, and more intensive case management strategies. Effective transitional care processes, linked with strong home care programs can reduce re-hospitalization by a third in some less intensive models and by half or more in some more intensive models.

Veteran's Affairs Home Based Primary Care

Julie Leftwich Beales and Thomas Edes

In response to the anticipated growth of the veteran population with chronic disabling diseases, the Department of Veterans Affairs (VA) established Home Based Primary Care (HBPC). This article focuses on that program, a home care program that specifically targets individuals with complex chronic disabling disease, with the goal of maximizing the independence of the patient and reducing preventable emergency room visits and hospitalizations. HBPC programs provide comprehensive longitudinal primary care by an interdisciplinary team in the homes of veterans with complex chronic disease, who are not effectively managed by routine clinic-based care. HBPC is very different from and complementary to standard skilled home care services, in population, processes and outcomes. HBPC targets persons with advanced chronic disease, rather than remediable conditions. HBPC provides comprehensive care of multiple co-morbidities, rather than problem-focused care. HBPC is delivered by an interdisciplinary team, rather than one or two independent providers. Currently operating in three-fourths of VA facilities, HBPC expansion continues to be driven by clinical success and the highest satisfaction of all VA services. VA HBPC is a model to emulate for the care of persons with complex, chronic disabling conditions, improving quality without added cost, and maximizing their independence through comprehensive longitudinal interdisciplinary care delivered in their homes.

K. Eric DeJonge, George Taler, and Peter A. Boling

By most clinical and economic measures, our health care system is not providing effective or affordable care to Medicare beneficiaries with severe chronic illness. Two million elders, constituting most of the 5% who account for nearly half of Medicare costs, have multiple chronic conditions, functional disability, and average per capita costs of over $50,000 per year. Prior reforms aimed at this population did not change the flawed delivery system, which remains centered in the doctor's office, hospitals, and nursing homes. This article describes a model of coordinated home-based medical care, called Independence at Home (IAH), which operates on a limited basis in many US communities and in the Veterans Affairs system. IAH-type teams deliver a full range of medical and social services at home to seriously ill elders and thereby reduce overall health care costs. We review the evidence that this approach can lower total costs by 25 percent or more while improving patient satisfaction and outcomes. We discuss funding for the new model, which also produces net savings for Medicare. A Medicare reform bill, called the Independence at Home Act, was introduced in the US House and Senate in 2008 to promote replication of this mobile elder care model.

THE CLINICS ARE NOW AVAILABLE ONLINE!

Access your subscription at:
www.theclinics.com

Preface

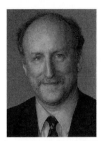

Peter A. Boling, MD
Guest Editor

Serving several million people each year in the United States with services ranging from high-touch basic support to high-tech medical therapy, home care helps individuals obtain their best possible function and remain where they prefer to be: at home. This edition of *Clinics* will review the origins of contemporary home care, beginning with parish nurses and doctors on horseback at the turn of the twentieth century and continuing through present-day care, which includes ventilators the size of a toaster oven, intravenous therapy, "smart houses," advanced information technology, and more. Each article has current, practical information, references regarding services and coverage, and reviews key evidence regarding impact. The authors articulate the building blocks for a future with fully elaborated, advanced models of care at home and conclude with a vision of that future.

In this review of home care, we will exclude normally ambulatory persons who use health care technology at home, like devices to self-manage illnesses such as diabetes, asthma, and hypertension, and tools to interact with health care providers. We will include people with functional limitations who are normally mobile and independent because of adaptive technology, such as otherwise healthy persons with paraplegia equipped with appropriate wheelchairs, ramps, elevators, and vans. These people require costly devices and supplies, plus home-health services when complications ensue, but not ongoing supportive care or case management. On the far end of the morbidity spectrum are those who are bedfast and completely dependent. Intermixed are persons of all ages with degrees of chronic illness burden and an enormous variety of conditions, short- and long-term care needs, upward and declining trajectories, those who are recovering and those who are dying. They share a common bond: the central locus of care is their home.

POPULATION NEED

Our best sources of insight are population-based surveys.[1] Varied methods affect the results, which in turn impact costs and resources, but the overall picture is clear and consistent. The 2003 National Health Interview Survey confirms that need for daily personal care rises sharply from age 65: 3% in men aged 65 to 74, 6% if aged 75 to

Clin Geriatr Med 25 (2009) xi–xiii
doi:10.1016/j.cger.2008.12.001
0749-0690/08/$ – see front matter © 2009 Elsevier Inc. All rights reserved.
geriatric.theclinics.com

84, and 17% if aged 85 or more. For women, the numbers are 3%, 7%, and 25%, respectively. About 3% of people need help getting around inside the home, with no change in the past decade, and about 3% of those aged 65 or more are unable to sit or get in or out of bed and chair without help. The 2005 Medicare Current Beneficiary Survey reports that 12% of aged community-dwellers need help getting out of bed or chair and 2% need help to eat. In the Longitudinal Study on Aging, 7% to 8% of community-dwellers have difficulty getting from bed to chair or leaving home. These people need a lot of help. For comparison, 70% of 2 million United States nursing home residents have such severe functional impairment.

There is some hopeful news: Medicare Current Beneficiary Surveys in 1992 and 2005 show a 3% decline in community-dwellers with deficits in instrumental activities of daily living and about the same numeric improvement in those having between three and six deficits in activities of daily living; yet, 7% still had such high-grade debility. While the modest decline in dependency is encouraging, there is a compelling consistency in the overall picture of need, and the decreasing incidence of disability is rapidly being eclipsed by the numeric growth in the aged population.

Community-dwellers with high-grade functional impairment (unable to sit, eat, transfer, or leave home without help) constitute only 2% to 7% of the elderly, but with about 40 million elders this subgroup currently numbers between 1 and 3 million people. In 15 years there will be at least twice this many. Because the segment aged 85 and over is growing even faster, the number of frail persons is likely to be at the upper end of that range, as the old-old have much higher rates of functional dependence.

HOME CARE USE AND EXPENSES

In all, home care accounted for only 2.4% of national health care spending in 2005, when hospital care consumed 31%, physician services 21%, drugs 10%, and nursing homes 6%. In 2004,[2] the average Medicare beneficiary had health care costs of $12,300, of which $375 involved home health care. Persons with three to six activities of daily living deficits consumed $31,631, with $1,386 spent on home health care.

Home care patients are complex: heterogeneity and comorbidity are typical. Though diseases such as congestive heart failure and diabetes have attracted attention from those interested in managing single diseases, these single diseases are the primary diagnoses for fewer than 10% of Medicare hospitalizations and Medicare home health care episodes. Home care patients carry many disorders, both common and rare.

The Congressional Budget Office projects growth in home-care expenditures (Parts A and B combined) from $15.5 billion in 2007 to $40.3 billion in 2018, while hospital inpatient care rises from $130 billion to $225 billion, Part D expenses rise from $49 billion to $138 billion, Medicare nursing home expenses grow from $22 billion to $40 billion, and hospice care increases from $10 billion to $21 billion.[2] Medicaid long-term care will grow from $57 billion to $139 billion. The Institute of Medicine in its report, "Retooling the Workforce for an Aging America," reported that in 2040 about 5 million elders would be receiving paid or formal long-term home health care services.

VALUE AND OPPORTUNITY

There is widespread awareness now that care of people with advanced chronic illness drives most of health care costs. Medicare beneficiaries with five or more chronic conditions consumed 66% of the 1999 Medicare budget. In 2005, The Congressional Budget Office confirmed that when beneficiaries are ordered by annual expense, the top 5%

use 43% of the budget, costing $63,000 each, and the next 5% use 18%, costing $27,000 each compared with the average at $7,300. Those who are high cost in the index year and live for 5 years are "high cost" users in 22 out of 60 months, revealing a pattern of relapsing and remitting acuity.

Counting all health care costs and dividing by population, average annual per capita expense to extend life 1 year for people aged 65 and over is about $145,000 in 2002 dollars.[3] Yet despite the spending, the United States ranks forty-fifth among nations in life expectancy in the 2008 World Fact Book of the United States Central Intelligence Agency.

Importantly, many persons with functional impairment and high chronic illness burden have preventable hospitalizations, and suffer from fragmented care that is far from patient-centered. This must be part of the explanation for the marked variation in average cost by state and region, while outcomes correlate poorly with the amount expended per capita.[4] Of special note is the frequency of hospitalization within the first 60 days of Medicare Part A home health care, which has remained constant or slowly rising near 28%. Half of these hospitalizations occur in the first 2 weeks, so that 7% of all users are hospitalized within 2 weeks, attesting to medical instability. Again, there is marked variation between agencies after case-mix adjustment.

Authors in this edition will show an increasingly persuasive array of studies that have demonstrated improved care with lower costs when implementing targeted, well-designed home-care interventions.

SUMMARY

Taken together, these findings define a growing population in need of home care, a large extant workforce with advancing technologic capabilities, and a currently fragmented, dysfunctional, costly model of care. An open mind enables one to envision the obverse of the current structure, which is centered on institutions like hospitals, nursing homes, and physician offices. Imagination, commitment, and perseverance are all that we need to transform health care and make the home the center rather than the periphery of our conceptual design. We foresee a truly patient-centered medical home.

Peter A. Boling, MD
Department of Medicine
Virginia Commonwealth University
PO Box 980102
Richmond, VA 23298, USA

E-mail address:
pboling@mcvh-vcu.edu

REFERENCES

1. Trends in Health and Aging. Available at: http://www.cdc.gov/nchs/agingact.htm. Accessed July 20, 2008.
2. CBO's March 2008 baseline: Medicare. Available at: http://www.cbo.gov/budget/factsheets/2008b/medicare.pdf. Accessed July 20, 2008.
3. Cutler DM, Rosen AB, Vijan S. The value of medical spending in the United States. New Engl J Med 2006;355(9):920–7.
4. Wennberg JE, Fisher ES, Goodman DC, et al. Tracking the care of patients with severe chronic illness. The Dartmouth Atlas of Health Care 2008. Available at: http://www.dartmouthatlas.org/atlases/2008_Chronic_Care_Atlas.pdf. Accessed January 16, 2009.

The Past, Present, and Future of Skilled Home Health Agency Care

Rachel L. Murkofsky, MD, MPH[a],*, Karen Alston, RN, MSN, MBA[b]

KEYWORDS

- Home care • Home health care • Home health agency
- Visiting nurse services • Skilled nursing services
- Skilled home health care

HOME HEALTH CARE IN THE UNITED STATES: BEGINNINGS TO PRESENT DAY
Beginnings of Home Health Care in the United States

The first documented home health care in the United States dates back to 1813, when the wealthy women of Charleston, South Carolina's "Ladies Benevolent Society," visited poor, sick patients in their homes to provide care and comfort. By the turn of the twentieth century, as a result of urbanization, industrialization, and immigration, American cities were dirty, crowded, and full of highly contagious, infectious diseases. There was a clear link between poverty and illness and a great motivation to protect society from uncontrolled disease. A small number of wealthy women in large cities, such as New York, Boston, Philadelphia, Buffalo, and Chicago, hired nurses to bring "care, cleanliness, and character" to the sick poor at home. Most of this care was provided free.[1,2]

Over time, the demand for these nurses grew. By 1909, almost 600 community organizations across the United States, including women's clubs, churches, hospitals, charitable organizations, health departments, and settlement houses, were sponsoring visiting nurses to protect the public from the spread of disease. That year Lillian Wald, who coined the phrase "public health nurse" and started the Henry Street Nurses Settlement House in New York City, convinced the Metropolitan Life Insurance Company to pay for the first visiting nurse benefit for sick policyholders in New York. By 1911, the company had extended its nursing services across the country and established the first national system of insurance for home care.[1,2]

[a] Department of Geriatric Medicine, John A. Burns School of Medicine, 347 North Kuakini Street, HPM-9, Honolulu, HI 96817, USA
[b] The Visiting Nurse Association of Greater Philadelphia, Monroe Office Center, One Winding Drive, Philadelphia, PA 19131, USA
* Corresponding author.
E-mail address: rmurkofs@hawaii.edu (R.L. Murkofsky).

Clin Geriatr Med 25 (2009) 1–17
doi:10.1016/j.cger.2008.11.006
0749-0690/08/$ – see front matter © 2009 Elsevier Inc. All rights reserved.
geriatric.theclinics.com

In the 1930s, hospitals began caring for patients with acute illnesses from all socio-economic groups, and visiting nurses began seeing patients with chronic illnesses. By the late 1950s, hospitals were routinely making referrals to home care nurses to facilitate discharge of their patients.[1] Home health agencies relied on charity and public contributions for the most part until the passage of the Medicare Act in 1965.[3]

Medicare and Home Health Care

In 1965, Medicare was signed into law as Title XVIII of the Social Security Act and extended health care coverage including home health care to nearly all Americans aged 65 years and older, regardless of income. Federal funding for home care not only provided much needed income for home health agencies but also regulated the benefit. It is often stated that home care was originally designed as a short-term, acute care benefit and that chronically ill patients were expected to manage at home with informal support from family, friends, or neighbors.[1] There were originally two distinct home health benefits: a post-hospital home health benefit under Part A (limited to 100 visits following a 3-day hospital stay) and a general home health benefit under Part B (limited to 100 home visits per calendar year). The Code of Federal Regulations at 42 CFR 409.44 clarifies the extent of the home health benefit at section b.3.iii: "The determination of whether skilled nursing care is reasonable and necessary must be based solely upon the beneficiary's unique condition and individual needs, without regard to whether the illness or injury is acute, chronic, terminal, or expected to last a long time."[4]

In 1967, there were 1,753 participating Medicare-certified home health agencies in the United States; by 1980, the number grew to 2,924.[5] Over the ensuing years, several legislative, judicial, and regulatory changes led to expanded eligibility criteria for home health care and increased demand for services.[1,6]

The Omnibus Reconciliation Act of 1980[7] removed limits on the number of home care visits, prior hospitalization requirements, and deductibles and extended participation in Medicare home care to for-profit home health agencies. In the late 1980s, the definitions of eligibility for home care were broadened as a result of Duggan v. Bowen.[8] Finally, the hospital prospective payment system (PPS) was implemented in the 1980s so that patients were discharged from the hospital "quicker and sicker."[9] As a result of these changes, there was an exponential growth in the number of agencies and patients plus Medicare home care expenditures (**Fig. 1A–D**). By the 1990s, the majority of Medicare home health episodes extended past 6 months: 37% lasted 6 to 11 months, and 24% lasted 12 months or longer.[10]

In 1997, there were 10,444 Medicare-certified home health agencies in the United States.[5] Fee-for service reimbursement created financial incentives for longer stays and more visits. Between 1990 and 1996, Medicare's home health expenditures increased by 350%.[11] Tremendous industry growth paralleled public reports of fraud and abuse.[12] In 1995, project Operation Restore Trust was implemented to identify fraud and abuse in home health care.[13]

The 1997 BBA and Home Health Care: Home Health Interim Payment System and Prospective Payment System

With the 1997 BBA,[14] Congress required the Medicare administration to develop a home health prospective payment system (PPS)[14] and control Medicare spending. At the same time, the Health Care Financing Administration began stricter enforcement of eligibility criteria for home care.[15] In addition, the BBA clarified the definition of part time or intermittent nursing care, required that the definition of "homebound" be studied, and excluded venipuncture as a sole eligibility criterion for skilled nursing services in home health care.[14]

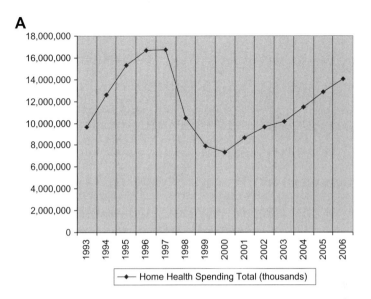

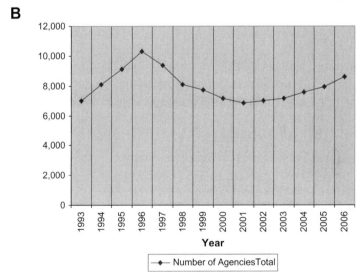

Fig. 1. Home Health Care from 1993 to 2006, *A.* Home health Spending, *B.* Number of home health agencies, *C.* Number of home care patients, *D.* Number of Medicare fee-for service enrollees. Data provided by the National Association for Home Care & Hospice: Data for spending and home health beneficiaries were extracted from the CMS Health Care Information System data set. The number of home health agencies was taken from the Online Survey, Certification, and Reporting data set provided by CMS. The number of Medicare enrollees was taken from CMS Medicare Enrollment Reports.

A home health Interim Payment System (IPS)[16] was implemented on October 1, 1997 to immediately curtail spending, while PPS was developed for initiation on October 1, 2000. In 1997, the IPS paid the least of an agency's actual costs, a reduced aggregate per-visit cost limit (decreased from 112% of average per-visit costs to 105% of median per-visit costs), or a new agency-specific per beneficiary limit based

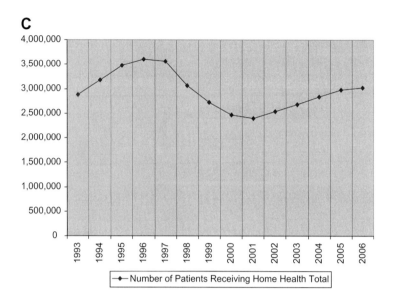

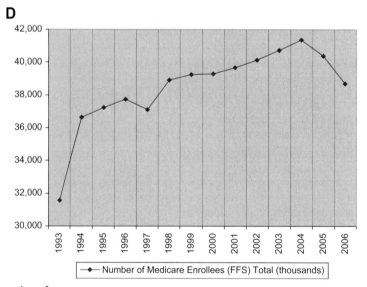

Fig. 1. (*continued*).

on 1994 costs.[14,16] PPS went into effect on October 1, 2000, and a further 15% cut in PPS payments took effect on October 1, 2002.[17]

Home health PPS was introduced with the intention of creating financial incentives for more efficient care. Under PPS, agencies are paid a set amount for each 60-day episode, regardless of the number of visits provided. Payments are case-mix adjusted, so agencies receive higher payments for complex patients. There are outlier payments for the care of the costliest beneficiaries and a per-visit payment for beneficiaries who require 4 or fewer visits during the 60-day episode. There are payment adjustments for those who require readmission to the same home health agency and for those who change home health agencies.[18] Until January 2008, adjustments were also made when beneficiaries experienced a significant change in their condition during an episode of care.[19]

With PPS, agencies are also required to obtain and report outcome data on all Medicare and Medicaid patients using the Outcome and Assessment Information Set (OASIS).[20] Although primarily designed for quality improvement as described below, selected OASIS items are used to define case-mix payments for the 60-day episode.

Effects of IPS and PPS

The Congressional Budget Office projected savings from the new home care reimbursement system of $16.2 billion during 5 years (1998–2002).[21] However, actual funding cuts under IPS were far larger than those anticipated,[22,23] which placed many agencies in financial jeopardy and caused changes in practice and service delivery. By 2001, more than one-third of US home health agencies had closed.[5]

Use of home care services

All studies of the impact of the 1997 BBA on home care found a marked decrease in utilization, with fewer Medicare beneficiaries receiving home care,[24–29] fewer visits per beneficiary,[24–28] lower payments,[26,29,30] and shorter care duration.[26,31–34] Declines in numbers of beneficiaries served and Medicare spending were consistent during both IPS and PPS. However, under PPS there was an increase in average payment per-visit,[28] likely due to both case-mix adjustment and agencies reducing visits per user. Agencies found case-mix adjusted PPS payments to be more predictable and sustainable than the drastically cut payments during IPS and started to recover.

Differential decreases in services were found for subsets of at risk elderly beneficiaries[24] aged 85 years and older,[26,27] living in states with high historical Medicare home health use,[27] using Medicaid or state assistance,[24,27] poor,[30] non-white,[27] female,[24,27] sick,[31] served by for-profit agencies,[24,27,34] first discharged to a skilled nursing facility or rehabilitation hospital,[24] and those with diabetes, heart failure, cerebrovascular disease, and skin ulcers.[27]

Outcomes of care

Although several studies evaluated decline in utilization of services using nearly identical measures, other outcome studies used disparate measures including post-home care utilization,[35] patient satisfaction with agencies,[36] pressure ulcer care,[37] and others derived from OASIS data.[38] Clinical outcomes improved for some conditions[38] and declined for others.[37,38] Satisfaction remained static for some, but others reported decreased satisfaction with some aspects of care.[36]

One study found that the types of patients receiving home care changed,[39] and many found changes in the mix of services, with dramatically fewer home health aide visits and fewer therapy visits.[27,29,31] These changes resulted from home health agencies altering behavior to function under PPS payment.

Over time, as agencies have adjusted to PPS, there has been a gradual increase in the number of home health agencies, the number of home care patients, and average payments (see **Fig. 1**A–C). In 2007, there were 9,284 Medicare-certified home health agencies in the United States, and Medicare spent more than $14 billion on home care.[5]

Medicaid and Home Health Care

The Medicaid program was created at the same time as Medicare in 1965. While Medicare extended health care coverage to nearly all Americans aged 65 years and older,

Medicaid provided health care services to people who were both poor and unable to work and included long-term supportive care. As the Medicare home care benefit was transformed by the BBA, many states expanded Medicaid home care programs.

The Medicaid expansion in home care services was motivated by an economic need to reduce nursing home expenditures; the Olmstead decision by the US Supreme Court in 1999,[40] which mandates provision of community alternatives to institutionalization for people with disabilities; and the federal New Freedom Initiative, which encourages states to provide community-based services. Between 1996 and 1999, Medicaid's share of home care spending grew from 17% to 33%.[41]

OASIS, Outcome-Based Quality Improvement, and the Home Health Quality Initiative

The Centers for Medicare and Medicaid Services (CMS) created the OASIS database for all US home health agencies. OASIS is a standardized comprehensive assessment for adult home care patients. Built during 10 years of development and formal testing, OASIS provides sociodemographic, environmental, support system, health status, and functional status data.[20]

Outcome-Based Quality Improvement (OBQI)[42] is CMS's systematic approach to help home health agencies improve the quality of care they provide. OBQI tracks and reports 41 risk-adjusted patient outcome measures that are based on OASIS data. OBQI reports are regularly provided to agencies to enable continuous quality improvement. Demonstration trials have shown that it is feasible to integrate OBQI into day-to-day operations of home health agencies, leading to outcome improvements.[43]

CMS now publicly reports 12 of the Home Health Quality Measures for each individual agency on the Home Health Compare Web site at www.medicare.gov (**Table 1**). New quality data are posted quarterly. Home Health Compare allows consumers and referring providers to see how well individual home health agencies are doing in assisting patients to regain or maintain function, review measures that are most important to them, and make comparisons between agencies.

Medicare Quality Improvement: The 9th Scope of Work

In August 2008, contracts were awarded for the 9th scope of work[44] of the Medicare Quality Improvement Organization (QIO) program, which focuses on improving the

| Table 1 |
| Home health compare quality Measures |

Quality Measure
Percentage of patients who get better at walking or moving around
Percentage of patients who get better at getting in and out of bed
Percentage of patients who have less pain when moving around
Percentage of patients whose bladder control improves
Percentage of patients who get better at bathing
Percentage of patients who get better at taking their medicines correctly (by mouth)
Percentage of patients who are short of breath less often
Percentage of patients who stay at home after an episode of home health care ends
Percentage of patients whose wounds improved or healed after an operation
Percentage of patients who had to be admitted to the hospital
Percentage of patients who need urgent, unplanned medical care
Percentage of patients who need unplanned medical care related to a wound that is new, is worse, or has become infected

Data from Centers for Medicare and Medicaid Services. Home Health Compare. U.S. Department of Health and Human Services, Baltimore, MD.

quality and safety of health care services to Medicare beneficiaries and is described in detail (in "The History of Quality Measurement in Home Health Care" article) by Rosati, elsewhere in this issue. National themes of the 9th scope include beneficiary protection, patient safety, and prevention. Targeted projects include diabetes disparities, care transitions, and chronic kidney disease prevention. QIOs will work in 14 states to coordinate care and promote seamless transitions across settings (hospital to home, skilled nursing, or home health care). QIOs will also seek to reduce avoidable hospital readmissions that increase both patient risk and Medicare costs. As of November 2008, 316 home health agencies have signed up with QIOs to participate in transition projects. Elderly patients who suffer adverse outcomes such as hospitalization are more likely to experience irreversible functional and health declines and poorer quality of life than patients who do not experience these events.[45–47]

HOME HEALTH CARE IN 2008
Goals of Home Care

The overall goal of home care is to provide treatment for an illness or injury and to help patients regain their independence and become as self-sufficient as possible. For long-term health problems, the goal of home care is to maintain the highest level of ability or health and learning to live with the illness or disability.

Many treatments provided in hospitals can also be done at home. When technically feasible, care given at home is usually less expensive and more convenient than care in a hospital or nursing home. With new technologies and pharmaceutical advances combined with a patient's desire to remain home, home care is preferred over emergency room care, hospitalization, or nursing home care.[48]

Home Health Payment Source

Home care service delivery is highly influenced by the payer source. Medicare is the single largest payer in home care. According to CMS,[49] sources for home health payment in 2006 were as follows: Medicare (37%), state and local government (19.9%), Medicaid (19%), private insurance (12%), and out of pocket (10%). Since the 1980s, shift in payer sources from traditional Medicare to managed care plans has presented challenges for agencies as they navigate the maze of payers' complex requirements. Some payers such as Medicaid and state and local funding offer greater flexibility, because they cover nonskilled and supportive services and may not require all patients to be homebound. An experienced, attentive staff is needed to manage all of these systems and use them well.

While traditional Medicare reimburses for care needed to meet a patient's medical and social needs for a 60-day episode with payment based on patient acuity, Medicaid and managed care plans usually pay a fixed rate per-visit and often require preauthorization for each visit. Average Medicare payment for a 60-day episode in 2008 is $2,300 ranging from about $1,276 to $7,758, and average visits per episode are about 18.[50] Typical health plan per-visit payments range from $75 to $110.

Unlike Medicare, the managed care per-visit approach focuses initially on one specific care goal. For example, skilled nursing may be ordered to provide wound treatments. Most wound care patients need to have comorbidities addressed, such as nutrition, mobility, incontinence, or diabetic control; a task-oriented approach to the wound is ultimately less effective. It is vital to have capable advocacy by experienced home health nurses who are adept at identifying unmet skilled needs and communicating those to insurer's case managers, resulting in additional visits.

Eligibility for Medicare Home Health Care

To be eligible for Medicare home care services, beneficiaries must meet the following criteria: (1) home care must be medically necessary and supervised by the patient's physician; (2) care must require a registered nurse (RN), physical therapist, or speech-language pathologist; (3) nursing care must be part time or intermittent; and (4) the patient must be homebound, meaning that leaving home is a considerable and taxing effort (**Table 2**).

Nonmedical absences from the home must be infrequent and of short duration, and the patient generally relies on the assistance of another person or the use of an assistive device or requires special transportation. Going to the doctor, for dialysis or other medical appointments, and to church are acceptable. Other absences from the home are permitted if the absence is infrequent or brief (such as occasional trips to the barber, a walk around the block, or a drive; attendance at a family reunion, funeral, graduation, or other unique event) and considerable and taxing effort is evident.[51]

Home health care must be provided at the patient's residence, defined as wherever the patient makes his or her home. Home care services cannot be rendered at a hospital or skilled nursing facility, but patients who reside in assisted living facilities or other group or personal care homes are eligible for Medicare home care services, if other requirements are met[51] (see **Table 2**).

Medicare Covered Home Care Services

Medicare covered services include skilled nursing care, provided by an RN or a licensed practical nurse; physical, occupational, or speech therapy; medical social work; home health aide services; and medical supplies. Service types for each discipline are described in **Table 3**. Social work and aide services may be provided only if the beneficiary is receiving covered skilled services.

Medicare does not pay for 24-hour care at home; meal delivery; homemaker services, such as shopping, cleaning, and laundry, when these are the only services needed, and the services are not related to the plan of care (PoC); personal care given by home health aides when this is the only care needed; or services and supplies that are excluded from the Medicare program. In addition, during a Medicare home care episode, a bundled payment is made to the agency for all covered services; Medicare will not pay for therapy or medical supplies from other providers and suppliers during the episode.

Medicare Conditions of Participation

The Medicare Conditions of Participation (CoPs)[52] govern all aspects of Medicare-certified home care agency operations, from compliance with federal, state, and local

---

Table 2
Medicare skilled home health care eligibility requirements

1. Homebound
   a. Nonmedical absences from home are infrequent
   b. Leaves home with difficulty and/or help
   • Medical care and treatments not counted, including dialysis
   • May have infrequent or brief social absences, such as for church, hairdresser, barber, or a special family event
2. Home care is safe and feasible
3. Care is medically necessary and reasonable
4. Physician orders the care

Table 3 Skilled home health services	
Provider Type	**Services**
Nursing	Assessments
	Teaching and training: medications, disease process, diet, treatments, and procedures
	Treatments and procedures: wound care, ostomy care, tracheostomy care, catheter care, injections, venipuncture
	Bladder and bowel training
	Intravenous therapy
	Psychiatric nursing
Physical therapy	Home exercise plan
	Strengthening exercises
	Training: gait, balance, transfers
	Ultrasound and other treatments
Occupational therapy	ADL and IADL training
	Fitting of orthotics
	Self-help devices
	Therapeutic activities for psychiatric patients
Speech therapy	Speech disorders
	Language disorders
	Swallowing disorders
Medical social work	Long-term planning
	Accessing community resources
	Crisis counseling
	Individual and family counseling
Home health aide	Personal care: bathing, dressing, grooming, hair care, nail care, oral hygiene
	Incidental care: light housekeeping, laundry, changing bed linens, meal preparation

Abbreviations: ADL, Activities of daily living; IADL, Instrumental activities of daily living.

Data from Centers for Medicare and Medicaid Services. Medicare benefit policy manual. U.S. Department of Health and Human Services, Baltimore, MD.

laws to basic elements of care. The CoPs guide federal quality oversight. Other payers, including Medicaid and some managed care plans, require contract agencies to have Medicare certification. Agency oversight is contracted to state Departments of Health through surveys. Failure to meet the CoPs may result in deficiency citations with penalties up to and including home health certification revocation.

Referrals to Home Care

Anyone may refer a patient for home care; however, a licensed physician (medical doctor, osteopathic doctor, or podiatrist) must order and oversee home care services. On receiving a referral, the agency verifies insurance coverage, obtains visit authorization if required, and verifies that the patient is not receiving home care from another agency.

Not all referred patients meet Medicare eligibility criteria. For instance, a patient may not be homebound or may lack a skilled care need. Some patients lack a suitable home environment; possible safety issues include the home's structural condition, lack of needed utilities, or risky conditions, such as an impaired caregiver or unsafe neighborhood. Lack of a willing, able, and available caregiver may also preclude home care if the patient cannot safely manage his or her own care. When a patient is not admitted due to lack of a payer or unsuitability for home care, the clinician notifies the physician and referral source so that other care options can be found.

The Typical Home Care Episode

The initial evaluation visit must occur within 48 hours (Medicare CoP) and must be completed by an RN unless the patient is to receive only physical or speech therapy. A typical admission visit may last 45 to 90 minutes. The admitting clinician determines eligibility, obtains consent for care, establishes the patient's financial responsibility, and presents the patient with required documents, such as advance directive information, privacy notices, and patient rights and responsibilities.

During the comprehensive initial assessment, the clinician collects the OASIS data, completes a medication review, and provides basic teaching and instructions to ensure patient safety until the next visit. Teaching is specifically related to the patient's diagnosis and immediate needs. For example, when admitting a new insulin-dependent diabetic, the RN assists the patient with preparing and administering insulin, teaches use of the glucometer, provides a written medication schedule, and instructs the patient on signs and symptoms of hypoglycemia and treatment, when to seek emergency care, and how to reach the on-call nurse. In this case, the nurse would likely visit again the next day. Frequency of subsequent visits is based on patient need.

Home care needs are identified during the comprehensive assessment. The admitting clinician designs a care path and prepares a 60-day (PoC) that describes all services (number of visits, medications, treatments) and establishes patient-focused goals. This PoC is verified and signed by the physician. Following the admission visit, each skilled discipline completes a discipline-specific evaluation and discipline-specific path and updates the treatment plan with new orders to be signed by the physician. During subsequent visits, each discipline works to reach the PoC goals.

Discharge planning begins at the start of care and is addressed throughout the course. As long as the patient needs skilled care, the agency can continue providing Medicare reimbursable services; rarely, this extends for years of sequential 60-day episodes, and agencies are under scrutiny to document necessity. Patients and caregivers are informed as individual goals are met, and a projected discharge date is identified. Patients actively participate in care planning. Ideally, the patient is discharged when the defined goals for home care have been met, although the patient may still be chronically ill and functionally limited. Some discharges result from noncompliance, patients no longer meeting Medicare criteria (eg, not homebound), or patients refusing further service.

Physician's Role in Skilled Home Health Agency Care

Home care requires an interdisciplinary team approach including the patient's physician. Although there often is no face-to-face contact by home care team members, Medicare CoPs require ongoing communication to coordinate care. Agency staff and patients need 24-hour access to the physician and prompt responses to telephone calls. Home health clinicians are required to report changes in patient status and are not allowed to prescribe treatments. The recent increase in physician home visits also signals a positive trend, since there is no equivalent substitute for firsthand involvement. A timely response to written communication is equally important, because signed physician's orders are required for every aspect of care, and payment may not be requested until all orders are signed.[48] Only a physician may sign home care orders for services provided by a Medicare-certified agency. Federal regulations prohibit nurse practitioners (NPs) from ordering home care despite recent state legis-lation that permits NPs to sign other care orders.

Referral to Hospice

When a patient has a life-limiting illness, hospice may be more appropriate than home health care, and a choice must be made. Home health nurses may refer patients for hospice care after discussing hospice with the patient, caregivers, and physician. Hospice orders also require physician authorization. Many home health agencies now have hospice divisions that can create a smooth transition. Patient choice is the deciding factor. Losing touch with trusted aides or other home health agency staff who have been involved for months or years may cause patients to decline hospice.

FUTURE DIRECTIONS FOR HOME CARE

The home care industry faces fiscal challenges. CMS pay for-performance (P4P) demonstration projects are underway. Cuts to traditional Medicare home health fund-ing are expected along with growth of Medicare Advantage (MA) plans, which use less home care. There is also a major planned overhaul in Medicaid. Both Medicare and Medicaid face major forecasted deficits associated with the baby boom.[53] All health care sectors must also consider how best to support "charity" care for 47 million unin-sured Americans. Without a payer for nursing home care, when discharged from hospitals, such individuals often have little choice but home care. Under these pres-sures, providers and payers are shifting to a chronic disease management approach.[53] Home health providers must constantly evaluate quality and service delivery models and increasingly rely on technology to achieve operational efficiencies.

From 1965 to 2000, quantity of services was the main driver for reimbursement. With home health PPS, quality measures, and chronic disease payment models, quality of service and outcomes will increasingly drive reimbursement. In January 2008, seven states began a CMS P4P demonstration project. The goal is to evaluate the impact of financial incentives for home health agencies that achieve the best outcomes, or demonstrate the greatest improvement, on seven of the 12 Home Health Compare quality measures. Although P4P will not be officially developed until Congress passes legislation, CMS envisions a budget-neutral program that awards competitive bonuses to top performers based on outcomes and Medicare savings, whereas worse performers receive reduced compensation. Also under construction are tiered discounts on consumer co-payments based on selecting high-quality providers.[53]

Introduced in January 2008, PPS reform includes a 2.75% annual reduction in Medi-care home health payments more than 4 years in response to a progressive rise in average PPS payment that resulted from increased case-mix weights. CMS contends that increased payments are based on changes in agency scoring practices rather than changing patient needs. To further control Medicare spending, a freeze in annual inflation updates has been recommended by the Medicare Payment Advisory Commission (MedPAC).[54] MedPAC is an independent congressional agency estab-lished in 1997 to oversee Medicare expenditures and quality.

Medicaid is the largest payer for long-term care, and state budget challenges are driving initiatives to move patients from nursing homes into community-based care. This requires strategic use of home care. CMS granted $1.75 billion during 5 years for Medicaid home and community care in the "Money Follows the Person" project. Funds can be used for home care, home modifications, respite care, personal care, or assistive devices. In addition, CMS recently published a final rule for self-directed care under State Medicaid programs and proposed new rules for redesigning Medicaid, giving states flexibility in their own Medicaid programs.[55]

The fastest growing sectors in the rapidly changing home care marketplace are private duty, personal care aides, and palliative care.[53] People prefer to remain at home, but they still need help after their skilled needs have been met, and most payers including Medicare do not cover custodial care. If not covered by Medicaid, access to these services depends on personal finances, long-term care insurance, and state-funded programs that provide personal care for financially eligible consumers. Palliative care programs bridge between traditional home care and hospice care by offering pain management and relief from debilitating symptoms. To compete, skilled home care agencies are expanding product lines and partnering with hospitals, assisted living facilities, and community-based programs to support a full continuum of community services.[53]

Home-based chronic care is essential for managing chronic disease. As defined by the Disease Management Association of America,[56] a chronic care system coordinates health care interventions and communications for patient populations with conditions that require significant self-care efforts. Bodenheimer and colleagues developed a widely adopted chronic care model[57] that guides care of patients with chronic diseases. Although physicians direct chronic medical care, home health clinicians are favorably positioned to assist physicians with care coordination. As complex patients have been discharged from acute care facilities earlier, home care clinicians have gained vital expertise. It is necessary to coordinate care well and adhere to evidence-based practice to prevent unnecessary inpatient admissions.[58]

With the above noted fiscal challenges, adoption of technology has become essential for efficient operations.[59] Four categories of technology are worth mentioning here: point of care computing, electronic medical records (EMRs), telephony, and telehealth. Personal digital assistants provide medication databases, while laptop and tablet computers record assessment data, build clinical pathways, and document care.[60] Portable computer technology, integral to the EMR, offers many benefits including reduced medical errors, improved clinical efficiency and accuracy of documentation, improved coordination of services, enhanced communication, and access to patient historical data.[61] Mobile broadband wireless technology has greatly improved efficiency by eliminating travel to the agency office or clinician's home to synchronize data. In addition, wireless technology allows e-mail access, an excellent communication tool for clinicians on the go.

The fully developed EMR has revolutionary potential within an agency. However, the ultimate goal is to create a centralized patient health care record accessible to home health agencies, physicians, hospitals, and other providers.[62] A national system with flow of data throughout the care cycle would greatly augment quality of care.

Although not in widespread use, electronic interface capability exists to connect home health agencies and physician offices to facilitate electronic communication and timely signature of orders. However, there are many interface problems that make this option impractical in most care settings. Integration between the agency's information system and medical supply vendors facilitates reordering of supplies, such as those for wound care, via the clinician's point of care device with automatic entry of supplies on the patient's insurance claim. Field clinicians can also request visit authorization directly from payers, eliminating paper reports. Today's competitive, reimbursement-constrained environment requires innovative technology solutions to reduce costs while increasing quality of care.[59]

Telephony refers to use of the telephone to transmit information. Home care telephony systems allow home health aides to access an integrated database to document personal care activities and record time and attendance. The system may be accessed from the patient's telephone via a toll-free number whereby the aide can review the care plan and receive instructions from the primary care clinician or messages from the supervisor. Telephony creates operational efficiency by eliminating back-office visit data entry and reduces fraud and abuse by verification of presence in the home and real-time documentation of care before leaving the patient's home.[60]

Research supports the proposed benefits of home telehealth, which has emerged as a useful tool for managing acute and chronic illness and improving quality of life.[63] Approximately 8% of the top home health agencies use telehealth. Successful telehealth programs report lowered emergent care utilization and hospitalization for selected conditions, such as heart failure, plus increased patient involvement in care management and satisfaction.[64] Further research is needed for best use of this promising technology.[65]

In April 2008, Fazzi Associates[66] released the Philips National Study on the Future of Technology and Telehealth in Home Care, finding that only 17% of agencies use telehealth technology. Fazzi advises home care agencies to seek and invest in integrative technology solutions. Telehealth reduces service delivery costs by using remote monitoring in place of some visits, reducing mileage fees, and increasing nursing productivity, allowing a larger caseload.

Combining the comprehensive assessments now being conducted with strong information technology and a seasoned workforce will position home health agencies as a key resource as we collectively move to address the coming societal challenges.

Although the aging population and new technology present exciting opportunities, the realities of reimbursement challenges, including P4P and increasing MA penetration, will require creative responses in the near term. In an environment of intense competition, escalating costs, service quality expectations, and product line diversification, embracing technology and implementing cost-saving measures are crucial for clinical and financial viability.

SUMMARY

Use of home health services decreased markedly after the 1997 BBA, with a change in the types of patients receiving home care and the mix of home care services. Much of this dramatic transformation was probably appropriate, given the uncontrolled growth and potential for fraud and abuse in the system. However, although eliminating unnecessary services and increasing efficiency, the BBA also probably reduced access to necessary services with unintended consequences, particularly for vulnerable subgroups that are at risk of adverse events.

With the current Medicare PPS, home health agencies have financial incentives to provide fewer visits and discharge patients quickly. Although there has been some recovery in the numbers of agencies and home care patients since 1997, patients discharged from home care too soon might be at risk for preventable adverse outcomes. In addition, although beneficiaries who are considered too costly may be refused service, no studies have specifically looked at outcomes of beneficiaries who no longer have access to home care following the 1997 BBA. To better inform health care policy, further studies are needed to determine how the home care population has changed since 1997; how access, quality, and outcomes of care have changed; and what the ongoing impact is of the BBA on Medicare beneficiaries.

The entire structure of health care finance and delivery is undergoing rapid evolutionary change, driven by population needs and costs. The expected impact of the baby boom and the ability to compete in a global economy underpin an urgent need to import technology, information system innovation, and evidence-based practices to produce high-quality care and desired outcomes at the lowest overall cost. In the end, it should be remembered that skilled home health care can help support our aging population to age in place at home.

ACKNOWLEDGMENTS

The authors thank Peter Boling and Mary St. Pierre for their thoughtful feedback on earlier versions of this manuscript.

REFERENCES

1. Buhler-Wilkerson K. No place like home: a history of nursing and home care in the U.S. Home Healthc Nurse 2007;25(4):253–9.
2. Buhler-Wilkerson K. The call to the nurse: our history from 1893 to 1943. Visiting nurse service of New York. Available at: www.vnsny.org/mainsite/about/a_history_more.html. Accessed September 24, 2008.
3. Grindel-Waggoner M. Home care: a history of caring, a future of challenges. Medsurg Nurs 1999;8(2):118–20.
4. Centers for Medicare & Medicaid Services. Title 42-Public Health; Chapter IV-Centers for Medicare & Medicaid Services, Department of Health and Human Services; Part 409-Hospital Insurance Benefits: 409.44: Skilled services requirements. Available at: www.access.gpo.gov/nara/cfr/waisidx_02/42cfr409_02.html. Accessed November 16, 2008.
5. National Association for Home Care & Hospice; Basic statistics about home care 2008; Washington, DC. The National Association for Home Care & Hospice. Available at: www.nahc.org/facts/08HC_Stats.pdf. Accessed January 16, 2008.
6. Testimony on Reforming the Medicare Home Health Benefit by Bruce C. Vladeck, PhD Administrator. Health Care Financing Administration, US Department of Health and Human Services. Hearing before the House Commerce Committee, Subcommittee on Health and Environment; Washington, DC. U.S. Department of Health and Human Services. Available at: www.hhs.gov/asl/testify/t970305a.html Accessed January 16, 2009
7. Public Law 96-499, Omnibus Reconciliation Act of 1980.
8. Duggan v. Bowen. 691 F. Supp. 1487; 1988.
9. Kosecoff J, Kahn KL, Rogers WH, et al. Prospective payment system and impairment at discharge. The 'quicker-and-sicker' story revisited. JAMA 1990;264(15): 1980–3.
10. Welch HG, Wennberg DE, Welch WP. The use of Medicare home health care services. N Engl J Med 1996;335(5):324–9.
11. Office of Research, Development, and Information, Centers for Medicare & Medicaid Services. Program Information on Medicare, Medicaid, SCHIP, and other programs of the Centers for Medicare & Medicaid Services: Medicare Fee-for-Service Home Health Expenditures June 2002. Available at: www.cms.hhs.gov/TheChartSeries/downloads/sec3d_p.pdf. Accessed January 16, 2009.
12. Publication of OIG Special Fraud Alerts: home health fraud, and fraud and abuse in the provision of medical supplies to nursing facilities. Fed Regist 1995;60(154): 40847–51.
13. Results of the operation restore trust Audit of Medicare Home Health Services in California, Illinois, New York and Texas. In: US Department of Health and Human

Services, Office of Inspector General. Publication A-04-96-02121 Washington, DC: Department for Health and Human Services; 1997.

14. Public Law 105-33, The Balanced Budget Act of 1997.

15. Medicare and Home Health Care. Baltimore (MD): Health Care Financing Administration, US Department of Health and Human Services; November 2000. Publication No. HCFA-10969.

16. Interim Payment System for Home Health Agencies. Subcommittee on health, committee on ways and means, house of representatives. Washington, DC: United States General Accounting Office; 1998. p. 1–12.

17. Centers for Medicare & Medicaid Services. Medicare program; Update to the Prospective Payment System for Home Health Agencies for FY 2003. Fed Regist 2002;67(125):43616–29.

18. Centers for Medicare & Medicaid Services. Home Health PPS overview. Available at: www.cms.hhs.gov/HomeHealthPPS/01_overview.asp. Accessed September 24, 2008.

19. Centers for Medicare & Medicaid Services. Medicare Program; Home Health Prospective Payment System rate update for calendar year 2009. Fed Regist 2008;73(213):65351–84.

20. Centers for Medicare & Medicaid Services. OASIS Overview. 12/28/2005. Available at: www.cms.hhs.gov/OASIS. Accessed March 29, 2007.

21. CBO Memorandum: Budgetary Implications of the Balanced Budget Act of 1997. Washington, DC: Congressional Budget Office: December 1997. Available at: www.cbo.gov/ftpdocs/3xx/doc302/bba-97.pdf. Accessed January 16, 2009.

22. Testimony of Paul N. Van de Water, assistant director for budget analysis, Congressional Budget Office, on the impact of the Balanced Budget Act on the Medicare Fee-for-Service program. Hearings Before the Committee on Finance, United States Senate. 1st edition; 1999. Available at: www.cbo.gov/doc.cfm?index=1322&type=0. Accessed January 16, 2009.

23. Testimony of Dan L. Crippen, director, Congressional Budget Office, on the impact of the Balanced Budget Act on the Medicare Fee-for-Service program. Hearings Before the Committee on Commerce, US House of Representatives. 1st edition; 1999. Available at: www.cbo.gov/doc.cfm?index=1553&type=0. Accessed January 16, 2009.

24. FitzGerald JD, Mangione CM, Boscardin J, et al. Impact of changes in Medicare Home Health care reimbursement on month-to-month Home Health utilization between 1996 and 2001 for a national sample of patients undergoing orthopedic procedures. Med Care 2006;44(9):870–8.

25. Liu K, Long SK, Dowling K. Medicare interim payment system's impact on Medicare home health utilization. Health Care Financ Rev 2003;25(1):81–97.

26. McCall N, Komisar HL, Petersons A, et al. Medicare home health before and after the BBA. Health Aff (Millwood) 2001;20(3):189–98.

27. McCall N, Petersons A, Moore S, et al. Utilization of home health services before and after the Balanced Budget Act of 1997: what were the initial effects? Health Serv Res 2003;38(1 Pt 1):85–106.

28. Murtaugh CM, McCall N, Moore S, et al. Trends in Medicare home health care use: 1997–2001. Health Aff (Millwood) 2003;22(5):146–56.

29. Spector WD, Cohen JW, Pesis-Katz I. Home care before and after the Balanced Budget Act of 1997: shifts in financing and services. Gerontologist 2004;44(1):39–47.

30. Zhu CW. Effects of the balanced budget act on Medicare home health utilization. J Am Geriatr Soc 2004;52(6):989–94.

31. Grabowski DC, Stevenson DG, Huskamp HA, et al. The influence of Medicare home health payment incentives: does payer source matter? Inquiry 2006; 43(2):135–49.

32. Han B, Remsburg RE. Impact of the Medicare interim payment system on length of use in home care among patients with Medicare-only payment source. Home Health Care Serv Q 2005;24(4):65–79.

33. Han B, Remsburg RE, Lubitz J, et al. Payment source and length of use among home health agency discharges. Med Care 2004;42(11):1081–90.

34. Murkofsky RL, Phillips RS, McCarthy EP, et al. Length of stay in home care before and after the 1997 Balanced Budget Act. JAMA 2003;289(21):2841–8.

35. McCall N, Korb J, Petersons A, et al. Constraining Medicare home health reimbursement: what are the outcomes? Health Care Financ Rev 2002;24(2):57–76.

36. McCall N, Korb J, Petersons A, et al. Decreased home health use: does it decrease satisfaction? Med Care Res Rev 2004;61(1):64–88.

37. Eaton MK. The influence of a change in Medicare reimbursement on the effectiveness of stage III or greater decubitus ulcer home health nursing care. Policy Polit Nurs Pract 2005;6(1):39–50.

38. Schlenker RE, Powell MC, Goodrich GK. Initial home health outcomes under prospective payment. Health Serv Res 2005;40(1):177–93.

39. Anderson MA, Clarke MM, Helms LB, et al. Hospital readmission from home health care before and after prospective payment. J Nurs Scholarsh 2005;37(1):73–9.

40. Olmstead v. L.C. In: Supreme Court of the United States, ed. 527 US 581; 1999.

41. Buhler-Wilkerson K. Care of the chronically ill at home: an unresolved dilemma in health policy for the United States. Milbank Q 2007;85(4):611–39.

42. Centers for Medicare & Medicaid Services. Home Health Quality Initiatives: OASIS OBQI. 07/25/2008. Available at: www.cms.hhs.gov/HomeHealthQualityInits/16_HHQIOASISOBQI.asp. Accessed November 16, 2008.

43. Shaughnessy PW, Hittle DF, Crisler KS, et al. Improving patient outcomes of home health care: findings from two demonstration trials of outcome-based quality improvement. J Am Geriatr Soc 2002;50(8):1354–64.

44. Centers for Medicare & Medicaid Services. Medicare Program; Evaluation Criteria and Standards for Quality Improvement Program Contracts (9th Scope of Work). Fed Regist 2008;73(140):42352–5.

45. Creditor MC. Hazards of hospitalization of the elderly. Ann Intern Med 1993; 118(3):219–23.

46. Gillick MR, Serrell NA, Gillick LS. Adverse consequences of hospitalization in the elderly. Soc Sci Med 1982;16(10):1033–8.

47. Lefevre F, Feinglass J, Potts S, et al. Iatrogenic complications in high-risk, elderly patients. Arch Intern Med 1992;152(10):2074–80.

48. American Medical Association and American Academy of Home Care Physicians. Medical management of the home care patient: guidelines for physicians. 3rd edition. American Medical Association; 2007. Available at: www.ama-assn.org/ama1/pub/upload/mm/433/homecare.pdf. Accessed January 16, 2009.

49. Centers for Medicare & Medicaid Services. Office of the Actuary, National Health Care Expenditures Historical and Projections: 1965–2016. Available at: www.cms.hhs.gov. Accessed August 21, 2008.

50. National Association of Home Care. Devil is in the Details: the home health PPS reform, 2007.

51. Centers for Medicare & Medicaid Services. Medicare Benefit Policy Manual, Chapter 7-Home Health Services 2008. Presented at: NAHC conference; Philadelphia.

52. Centers for Medicare & Medicaid Services. Title 42-Public Health, Chapter IV-Health Care Financing Administration, Department of Health and Human Services, Part 484-conditions of participation: home health agencies. Available at: www.access.gpo.gov/nara/cfr/waisidx_99/42cfr484_99.html. Accessed January 5, 2006.

53. Remington L. Industry trends, forecasts and predictions: 2008 and beyond. Visiting Nurse Associations of America Annual Conference. Nashville, TN; 2008. Available at: www.cms.hhs.gov/manuals/Downloads/bp102c07.pdf. Accessed January 16, 2009.

54. Medicare Payment Advisory Commission. Report to the Congress: medicare payment policy; Section 2E: Home Health Services. Washington, DC; 2008: 171–87.

55. Centers for Medicare & Medicaid Services. 42 CFR Part 441: Medicaid Program; Self-Directed Personal Assistance Services Program State Plan Option (Cash and Counseling); Final Rule Vol 73; 2008:57854–86.

56. Disease Management Association of America. Population Health: DMAA definition of case management. Available at: www.dmma.org/dm_definition.asp. Accessed October 4, 2008.

57. Bodenheimer T, Wagner EH, Grumbach K. Improving primary care for patients with chronic illness: the chronic care model, Part 2. JAMA 2002;288(15):1909–14.

58. Suter P, Hennessey B, Harrison G, et al. Home-based chronic care. An expanded integrative model for home health professionals. Home Healthc Nurse 2008; 26(4):222–9.

59. Crownover K. The changing role of technology companies in home care and hospice. Caring 2008;27(7):40–2.

60. Waters RJ, Eder-van Hook J. Technology essential to effective home care administration & patient care. Caring 2006;25(7):10–2, 14–7.

61. Trescone D. Success at the point of care. Caring 2006;25(7):40–2.

62. Feth B. Providing quality care while introducing new technology. Caring 2006; 25(7):36–8.

63. Meyer M, Kobb R, Ryan P. Virtually healthy: chronic disease management in the home. Disease Management 2002;5(2):87–94.

64. Conrad C, Fuller E, Kessler S. Telehealth: is it the silver bullet? Caring 2007;26(7): 26–32.

65. Bowles KH, Baugh AC. Applying research evidence to optimize telehomecare. J Cardiovasc Nurs 2007;22(1):5–15.

66. Fazzi Associates. Philips National Study on the Future of Technology & Telehealth in Home Care; 2007.

The Past, Present, and Future of House Calls

Helen Kao, MD[a], Rebecca Conant, MD[a], Theresa Soriano, MD, MPH[b],
Wayne McCormick, MD, MPH[c],*

KEYWORDS

- Homebound • Home care • Home health care
- House calls • Home visits • Home-based medical care

ORIGIN OF HOUSE CALLS

The classic image of a doctor up through the mid-20th century was that of a community physician, black bag in hand, traveling to a patient's home where he would provide care. Physician house calls were once the primary mode of health care delivery in the United States and Europe. Before World War II, every tool a physician had available to diagnose and treat a patient could be packed into the black bag. The practice of house calls was prevalent in this earlier era before most individuals lived in compact cities. Physicians were more likely than patients to have access to means of transportation, whether horse or automobile, making health care most efficiently delivered in the home by the traveling doctor.

EVOLUTION OVER TIME

During the 20th century, dramatic changes in health care affected the way health care was delivered. House calls dropped from 40% of physician encounters in 1930 to 10% by 1950 and less than 1% by 1980.[1,2] As the number of physicians making house calls fell, the nature of house calls also changed. Through the early 20th century, house calls were the primary mode of medical care. However, as technology, physician specialization, and payment systems changed, primary care moved into clinics, and house calls largely became a relic of the past. Primary care physicians focused on office encounters and rarely made home visits, generally doing so only to visit a long-term patient who had become too frail or homebound to come to the office.

[a] University of California, San Francisco, UCSF Box 1265, 3333 California Street, #380, San Francisco, CA 94118, USA
[b] Mount Sinai School of Medicine, New York, Mount Sinai Visiting Doctors Program, Box 1216, One Gustave Levy Place, New York, NY 10029, USA
[c] University of Washington, Harborview Medical Center, 325 9th Avenue 359755, Seattle, WA 98104, USA
* Corresponding author.
E-mail address: mccorm@u.washington.edu (W. McCormick).

Clin Geriatr Med 25 (2009) 19–34
doi:10.1016/j.cger.2008.10.005
0749-0690/08/$ – see front matter © 2009 Elsevier Inc. All rights reserved.

By the turn of the 21st century, physicians were divided into those who never or rarely made house calls and the few who continued to make regular house calls. In 2001, less than 18% of US physicians made house calls. Those physicians who did make house calls averaged 5 house calls per week.[3] The small cadre of physicians who have made house calls a major focus is so small that they are not well represented in these statistics. In contrast, most primary care physicians in Europe and Canada continue to make substantial numbers of house calls as a routine aspect of home and community-based care. Physicians in England make 10 times the number of house calls per 1,000 patients per year compared with US physicians and 100 times as many to persons older than 85 years.[4,5]

With the growing availability of medical and transportation technology, medical care became housed in medical institutions. Diagnostic and therapeutic technology required increasing space and maintenance, and specialization of practitioners was such that medical care came to be based in hospitals and clinics. Car ownership also became commonplace, and public transportation systems sprang up in urban centers enabling patients to visit physicians more easily. Physicians' specialization and subspecialization in medicine have also been greatly influenced by hospital-based diagnostic and therapeutic advances in technology.[6,7] The exceptions to this trend are geriatrics and palliative care. While many palliative care services remain hospital-based, the growth of home hospice programs supported by the Medicare hospice benefit has allowed many individuals to receive end-of-life care in their home. Likewise, geriatric specialists, by nature of caring for frail elders, have kept attention on access to care for homebound elders.

The economics of medical care has also influenced the decline of house calls. The growth of managed care and overhead burden created increasing pressure for "productivity" and forced primary care physicians to provide care as efficiently as possible—generally meaning abandoning house calls and exclusively practicing in clinics, pushing daily patient encounter volumes to the highest safe level to offset their overhead. Although there has been very little litigation in home care, concerns over medical liability also contributed to the shift of care from home to hospitals and clinics.[8] As more advanced technology was used for diagnosis and treatment of illness, physicians and patients alike came to expect high-technology medicine.[9] With this expectation was the association of "good medicine" with hospitals and clinics.[10] House calls became "old fashioned."

Physicians who do make house calls are now almost exclusively practicing in a primary care field providing comprehensive care. A survey of Virginia Medicaid providers found that physicians who make routine house calls to patients (compared with those who never or only emergently made house calls) were more likely to be family physicians than internists. Physicians who make house calls were more likely to use and collaborate with home health agencies. These physicians were also significantly more likely to consider the following as indications for home visits: chronic disease management, acute illness, end-of-life care, death pronouncement, difficulty transporting patient, and personal satisfaction from home visits.[11] Physicians often cite terminal care as a reason for making house calls.[11]

During this shift in primary care from home to office, the availability of Medicare-supported home health agencies has been vital. The growth of home health care agencies, discussed in an article by Murkofsky and colleagues, elsewhere in this issue, has helped improve health outcomes of homebound individuals. In the 1990s, skilled home health care was the fastest growing component of the Medicare budget.[12] Yet, while home health agency care has enabled homebound patients to live at home and recover there from serious illness, historically, there has been inadequate involvement of physicians in home care.[11] Most patients receiving skilled home care do not receive physician house calls as part of their care,[13] and active physician involvement in the care plan is limited.[14] Unlike hospices and nursing homes, home health agencies are not required to have a medical director. If one exists, the medical director is not required to make home visits, and most patients receiving home care must still travel to a physician's office for medical care. It is not surprising that for many house calls practices, new referrals often come from community home health agencies because house calls address a need not fulfilled by home health agencies alone and not met by office-based physicians.[15]

Concurrent with the institutionalization of medicine, the United States has stumbled into a primary care crisis. Fewer medical school graduates are choosing to specialize in general internal medicine, general pediatrics, and family medicine. Between 1995 and 2005, there was a 40% reduction in graduates entering family medicine and between 1998 and 2005, a 37% reduction in internal medicine residents who remained generalists. This primary care crisis further threatens the home medical care workforce. In the 1990s, generalists comprised 12% of physicians caring for adults but accounted for 87% of physicians providing house calls to the elderly.[4] Positions in family medicine residencies are unfilled every year.[16] If these trends continue, there will be a shortage of 44,000 adult care generalists by 2025.[17] The geriatrician workforce is even more seriously undermined, and that situation is not improving. In 2006–2007, only 54% of first-year geriatric fellowship spots were filled.[18]

There is an additional issue with poor preparation of the generalist workforce for home-based care. Medical schools and residency programs are considering how best to teach physicians to care for patients at home, and penetration of the curriculum is limited. In the 1990s, only 66 of 123 medical schools reported exposing students to more than 1 hour of home care curriculum, and only 3 schools required that their students go on more than 6 home visits.[19] Over the past 20 years, several mainstream health provider organizations have encouraged increased education and involvement of physicians in home care. These include the American Medical Association, American Geriatrics Society, American College of Physicians, and American Academy of Home Care Physicians.[15] The 2008 Institute of Medicine report[20] on the geriatric medicine workforce underlined this point, as discussed further by Hiyashi and colleagues, in an article elsewhere in this issue.

TRENDS IN SERVICE VOLUMES: THE PAST 40 YEARS AND THE RECENT RESURGENCE

The need for physician house calls will grow as the US population ages. The population of persons aged 65 years and older in the United States was 7% in 1940, was 12% in 2000, and is estimated to be 20% by 2030. Eleven percent (3.7 million) of older Medicare enrollees received personal care services in 1999. In 2006, nearly a third (10.7 million) of noninstitutionalized elders lived alone.[21] By 2020, an estimated 2 million elderly are expected to be homebound due to physical and cognitive impairments that make it difficult for them to leave their home.[22] Yet, through the 1980s into the 1990s, the number of physician house calls billed to Medicare declined by 31%. In 1993, Medicare reimbursements for physician house calls were substantially less than those for skilled nursing, physical therapy, speech therapy, or occupational therapy.[4]

Fortunately, in the past decade, house calls have experienced resurgence. In 1998, Medicare established new billing codes that better described home visits and increased reimbursements for physician house calls by nearly 50%. In 2001, reimbursement for visits to assisted living facilities similarly increased. Despite some reductions in payment since 2006, the number of house calls billed to Medicare has increased annually since the 1998 change. Although the total number of house calls remains less than 1% of all outpatient evaluation and management services billed to Medicare,[23] mobile visits have increased both in absolute number and in proportion. Medicare data show that physician house calls increased from 1.5 million in 2000 to almost 2.2 million in 2007. Domiciliary visits (assisted living and adult homes) have also grown, increasing from fewer than 1.6 million in 2006 to almost 1.8 million in 2007.[24] Between 1998 and 2003, geriatricians demonstrated the greatest growth in annual house calls amongst physicians, a proportionate increase of 92% compared with 41% for family practitioners and 59% for internists; family practitioners continue to make the greatest total number of house calls.[25] Podiatrists, psychiatrists, and surgeons made fewer house calls over the same time period.

During this decade of home visit resurgence, Medicare reimbursements for physician visits to homes and domiciliary facilities increased to a peak of $213 for complex new patient visits in 2005, and the value of the most commonly used code rose to around $100. An increasing number of physicians have chosen full-time house call practice as their preferred professional role. The growth of house calls has been fostered not only by Medicare payments but also by hospital-supported house calls programs, transitional care programs for early hospital discharge, and improved home visit curricula in medical education.[23,26] These favorable changes notwithstanding, adequacy of reimbursement is a significant factor and challenges remain: Medicare payments for house calls fell up to 20% between 2005 and 2008 and are expected to remain low through 2010.[27,28] In addition, as is true for all primary care services, thin margins and modest take-home pay make the choice of house call practice one that places the provider at the lower end of the physician pay scale.

WHAT THE PATIENT, FAMILY, AND PROVIDERS UNIQUELY GAIN FROM HOUSE CALLS COMPARED WITH ENCOUNTERS IN OTHER CARE SETTINGS

House calls offer many advantages to patients, families, and providers beyond what is obtained in the typical outpatient clinic or acute hospital setting. Providing primary care at home is not simply a "convenience" for an elderly patient who might find a trip to the doctor's office an overwhelming challenge, even with caregiver assistance and wheelchair or ambulance transport. For patients who are particularly frail or have severe mobility impairment, coordinating and executing a physician's office visit often carry both a financial price and substantial physical discomfort. Patients report that it takes days to recover from the experience. For patients with dementia or psychiatric disorders causing paranoia or behavioral disturbance, leaving home for a clinic visit may trigger psychological distress, and patients may simply refuse. Moreover, for patients in terminal stages of disease, the home is often the most appropriate and comfortable setting for care.[29]

Almost everything that is done in an office visit can now be accomplished at home with portable medical technology. In addition, with the support of home health agencies, many patients can safely receive treatment at home for acute illnesses that would otherwise result in an emergency room visit or acute hospitalization. Avoiding hospitalization saves more than money. Despite remarkable improvements in technical capability, hospitalization adds considerable risk of acquiring resistant bacterial infections and suffering iatrogenic complications, and it almost guarantees discontinuous medical professional care.

Aside from providing access to continuous, primary care for homebound elders, house calls improve patient care by clarifying and identifying problems that are missed in the clinic setting. In the home and domiciliary settings, the provider can see the patient as a person in his or her own environment and with the people involved in that individual's daily life. Exploring the patient's environment yields a wealth of new information that is both quantitative, such as previously missed diagnoses or discrepancies in medication regimens, and qualitative in terms of grasping what the person can do and what the support system can provide. A home visit can uncover illicit drug or alcohol abuse, environmental contributors to frequent falls, incontinence, and early signs of dementia or caregiver burnout, all of which may go unnoticed during an office visit.

Physicians who make house calls provide better coordination of care in conjunction with home health agencies. House calls physicians refer to skilled home health agencies and pharmacy delivery programs more often than physicians who are strictly clinic-based.[11] When physicians use home health agencies, those who make house calls are more likely to understand Medicare guidelines and to write more comprehensive orders than office-based colleagues. The home health care providers are then better able to tailor treatment to patient and physician goals.[15] In general, house call physicians are better prepared to partner with other home health providers due to their familiarity with home care in all of its dimensions, much as surgeons are more familiar with the operating room.

House calls physicians provide important care to patients whose needs extend beyond what is provided by home health agencies. House calls care is complementary to the work of agency staff. Patients may have complicated conditions or require a higher level of care than that provided by home health agency nurses, including wound debridement, new diagnoses, and adjusting complex medical regimens in response to changes in condition. Skilled home care is also generally brief and intermittent, whereas care needs of patients with complex medical comorbidities do not end when they are discharged by the home health agency. These patients need ongoing medical management for advanced chronic diseases. When patients become homebound, they often lose their primary medical care provider, either because the provider is unable or unwilling to make house calls or because the patient has had to move in with family for support and thus has had to relocate away from the former primary provider.[15] House calls ensure continuity of care.

Patients benefit from house calls by receiving the level of care they want in the setting they prefer. Homebound patients and their surrogates may decide at some point to avoid hospitalization. In addition to primary care, many house calls programs provide urgent care and even "hospital at home." One study of a house calls program found that over 2 years, 59% of patients experienced an acute illness or complaint requiring an urgent telephone call or in-home assessment. These conditions included many that might normally prompt an emergency room visit or hospitalization. Seventy-three percent of the acute problems were successfully evaluated at home and treatable with oral medications. Only 3 cases required hospitalization.[30] A recent study of home-based geriatric care for at-risk elderly also found reduced acute care use in the second year of a 2-year randomized controlled trial.[31]

Family and caregivers of patients receiving house calls are better integrated into a patient's comprehensive care plan. They have the advantage of improved on-site communication with physicians. If medications are adjusted or recommendations for lifestyle changes made, the physician and team nurse can provide hands-on education, including use of the patient's pill bottles, refrigerator, and kitchen cabinets as teaching tools. Families have peace of mind: not only is their loved one cared for despite becoming homebound but also the caregivers are not abandoned. By exploring the patient-caregiver relationship at home rather than the office, physicians are better able to see when caregivers need more support, education, or respite. For instance, for a woman who is immobilized by debility and cardiopulmonary disease, it may not be obvious in clinic that the patient's husband is unable to reposition her in bed or safely assist in transfers from bed to chair.

Physicians who make house calls frequently cite immense personal satisfaction from providing this type of care. They feel that they provide an important service and believe this service is needed regardless of available visiting nurses or transportation. They are more likely than physicians who never, or only occasionally, make house calls to feel that home visits are enjoyable, and they are less likely than occasional house callers to feel they are too busy to make house calls.[11] Medical school curricula teach students not only clinical indications for, but also the rewards of, providing care at home. Evaluations of medical students exposed to home visits with geriatricians show that the students have increased empathy and respect for patients with chronic illness. Home visits enable students to appreciate the rewards of helping frail older patients continue to lead full lives at home.[32]

KEY CLINICAL ISSUES IN THE HOME

Several key clinical issues are more effectively evaluated and addressed in the home setting than in the physician's office. While the topics discussed here are far from a comprehensive list of the problems physicians address during house calls, they comprise core clinical issues that significantly affect homebound patients' well-being.

Home Environment and Function

An obvious advantage of house calls is assessing the home environment and the patient's ability to function therein. Many patients are homebound due to gait instability and are at risk for falls; even a single fall can cause serious morbidity or death. A home visit permits a comprehensive assessment, which, when linked with the support of an interdisciplinary team of specialists, can reduce environmental hazards and improve the patient's ability to sit, transfer, and ambulate safely. Home visits for disability prevention improve gait and balance in individuals at low risk of nursing home placement; for individuals at high risk of institutional placement, rehabilitation together with care coordination is most effective.[33] Based on several studies, comprehensive geriatric assessment with multiple house calls (9 or more) is significantly associated with reduced functional decline, nursing home use, and mortality.

All members of an interdisciplinary team should notice and address environmental hazards such as rugs, cords, or hallways too cluttered for safe maneuvering. Physical and occupational therapists can best determine appropriate assistive devices, exercise programs, home adaptations, and footwear. The physician examines the patient for orthostasis, neuropathy, weakness, visual impairment, and other medical factors that impair functional and cognitive status. The physician and nurse can explore the home for nonprescription medications or inappropriately filled medication boxes that may lead to falls. Medical care providers, social workers, and therapists should watch for signs of surreptitious alcohol consumption, unsanitary conditions, or inadequately educated and overextended or neglectful caregivers who are unsure of how to safely assist the patient or are in need of more help.

The advantages of direct home assessments compared with office-based evaluations have been well established. Social and environmental problems identified by office-based physicians are rarely specific enough compared with home visit assessments to allow for development of effective treatment plans.[34] Additionally, when problems are identified by office-based assessments, the risk associated with these problems for patient and caregiver well-being is frequently underestimated.[35]

Skin Assessment

For patients who are minimally ambulatory or already limited to their chair or bed, house calls allow the physician to regularly conduct a thorough skin assessment and follow the progress of wound care with greater ease than in the office. Patients whose severe functional impairments place them at risk for skin breakdown are the same patients for whom climbing onto an examination table in an office may be nearly impossible and extremely time-consuming. In a busy clinic, the office-based physician often forgoes a full skin examination or relies on communications with visiting home health nurses about the status of wounds. During home visits, patients are either in bed or can be placed in bed before the physician's arrival. The physician can assess the skin, skin hygiene routine, wound dressing methods, and transfer techniques to correct caregiver practices that contribute to skin breakdown, irritation, or tearing.

Cognitive Assessment

Cognitive assessments and determination of decision-making capacity are critical components of home visits. The decision to remain living independently at home is made by many older patients but must be assessed within a larger framework to determine (1) if remaining at home is safe; (2) whether the individual has adequate caregiver support; and (3) if there are signs of self-neglect. One study of community-dwelling elderly patients referred to a geriatric home assessment program found that the most common reason for referral was memory difficulties and that more patients had probable dementia diagnoses than had hypertension.[34] Twenty-three percent of new problems identified during home visits, but not in comprehensive clinic-based evaluation, are psychobehavioral problems, such as depression, confusion, and agitation.[34] Finding cognitive impairment can prompt physicians to coordinate with interdisciplinary teams to establish financial representative payees, conservators, other psychobehavioral supports, and, if needed, to contact Adult Protective Services. Patients often perform better, and thus have more accurate evaluations, during home-based assessments in familiar settings than they do in the clinic.

End-of-Life Care

Progressive functional decline precluding travel becomes common as individuals approach the end of life. Patients with terminal processes, whether enrolled in a hospice or not, benefit from continuing care by a physician who can visit the patient at home. Terminal care and death pronouncement are among the indications for visits identified by physicians who make house calls.[11] Though physician visits are not needed frequently during most hospice care, there are times when an experienced physician can improve the care plan and provide reassurance to the patient and family that all needed care is being given. In fact, home visits outside of the hospice benefit can act as a bridge to hospice by providing cost-effective palliative care to patients who do not yet qualify for hospice or choose not to enroll, and they may increase subsequent hospice referral and reduce emergency room use and hospitalizations.[36,37] Physician comfort with the types of therapy shown in **Table 1** enhances the effect of visits made during terminal care.

Specific Medical Issues

In several clinical areas, there is unique medical knowledge specific to the home setting, which is requisite for effective home care practice. These areas include wound care, respiratory care and oxygen therapy, bladder and bowel management, enteric and intravenous feeding, intravenous therapy, use and coverage of durable medical

Table 1
Medication delivery modalities useful in a home setting

Modality	Examples	Indications	Result
Topical/Transdermal	Anesthetics (lidocaine)	Neuropathy, Post-herpetic neuralgia	Temporary, local pain relief
	Opioids (fentanyl)	Chronic stable pain, unable to take oral opioids	Sustained systemic pain relief
	Capsaicin	Neuropathy, Post-herpetic neuralgia	Temporary, local pain relief. Often burns on initial application until substance P is depleted.
	Anticholinergics (eg, scopolamine)	Excessive oropharyngeal secretions; nausea; visceral pain	Reduced oral and gut secretions
Thermal	Heat	Muscle spasm, chronic inflammation, joint stiffness/pain	Relax local muscles and increase blood flow
	Cold	Sprains, strains, inflammation	Reduce local edema and blood flow
Electrotherapy	Transcutaneous electrical nerve stimulation	Acute and chronic musculoskeletal pain, peripheral nerve injury	Muscle contraction and strengthening, increases circulation
Nebulized	Morphine	Dyspnea	Quick relief of dyspnea (controversial)
Subcutaneous infusion	Opioids	Pain, dyspnea	Quick onset pain relief, easily titrated to comfort
Sublingual	Liquid morphine, soluble morphine tablets	Dysphagia	Concentrated solutions are absorbed quickly for fast pain relief
	Benzodiazepines (eg, lorazepam, diazepam)	Anxiety related to dyspnea, agitation, nausea, opioid-related myoclonus	Anxiolytic and relief of myoclonus
Rectal	Acetaminophen	Pain, fever	Relief of pain and fever
	Neuroleptics (eg, chlorpromazine)	Nausea	Useful for opioid-related nausea
	Corticosteroids (eg, dexamethasone)	Pain, increased intracranial pressure, nausea	Reduce inflammation and intracranial swelling
	Anticonvulsants (eg, gabapentin, carbamazepine)	Neuropathic pain	Useful in patients unable to swallow

Data from McCleane G. Topical analgesic agents. Clin Geriatr Med; 24:299–312; and Schneider H, Cristian A. Role of rehabilitation medicine in the management of pain in older adults. Clin Geriatr Med; 24:313–34.

equipment and other assistive devices, and in-home diagnostics. To effectively manage acute problems, physicians must also know the best and most easily delivered treatment options, such as anti-infective therapy. Like palliative care and nursing home care, there is much to know about medications that can be delivered in liquid, aerosol, or topical forms, medications for behavior disturbances in dementia, and medications for delirium or pain (see **Table 1**).

Home Atmosphere

Finally, the interaction between provider and patient (and caregivers) is a fundamentally different dynamic in the patient's home. The home is the venue of daily life, where friends and family are in control and are comfortable. The physician enters this environment as a guest and helper and as a friend and confidant. One gains an appreciation of a loving and supportive environment, as contrasted with dangerous and often unhealthy institutional environments; this awareness usually escapes clinic providers but is immediately apparent during the house call.

EVIDENCE THAT HOUSE CALLS IMPROVE PROCESS OR OUTCOMES

It is a matter of common sense that house calls improve health care for homebound patients in several respects. At the most fundamental level, house calls provide access to care for millions of patients who are unable to visit physician offices, particularly at times when the patient most needs help. Urgent care might otherwise only be accessible in an emergency room and chronic care in a nursing home. Beyond simply providing homebound patients with access, there is growing evidence that house calls favorably influence important health outcomes. One is satisfaction with care, increasingly recognized as an important quality measure. In addition, evidence of benefit includes improved physical function and reduced nursing home use for certain subsets, reduced hospitalization, and reduced mortality when care is done right and patient selection is well targeted.

Multidimensional and interdisciplinary house calls practices prevent and reduce functional decline. One meta-analysis demonstrates that home visits reduce mortality and admission to long-term nursing home care for both general and frail elderly.[7] As mentioned here, this is probably because these programs identify new or worsening medical problems or social conditions that could lead to patient decline or death. In one study, home assessments uncovered at least 1 new problem in 72% of patients and 3 or more problems in nearly a quarter.[34] Another study comparing home visits to clinic-based assessments found that 95% of patients have at least 1 problem that was identified only by the home visit. When problems were identified both in clinic and at home, the clinic-based assessments consistently underestimated the risk associated with serious problems.[35] The dramatically improved detection of important health problems when patients are assessed at home rather than using a clinic-based approach was confirmed in the Gender, Race, and Clinical Experience (Geriatric Resources for Assessment and Care of Elders [GRACE]) study.[31]

As most individuals prefer to stay in their homes as they age, home-based geriatric assessments that improve function enable patients to live at home safely. Studies of community-dwelling older adults show that individuals randomized to receive geriatric home visits compared with control subjects maintain higher mean functional levels.[38,39] Patients in these individual studies required less assistance with activities of daily living and were less likely to be placed in nursing homes. One meta-analysis in 2001 found that improvement in function (specifically instrumental activities of daily living) occurred only for a general elderly population.[7] However, a study in 2002 using multidimensional assessments, with at least 9 follow-up home visits, found risk of functional decline reduced by 24%.[40]

House calls can also address social isolation and health care costs. Social isolation with difficulty accessing acute care is a significant risk factor for nursing home placement and dying at home alone.[41] As a result of the comprehensive nature of home-based interventions, seniors are more likely to be connected to adult education or friendly visitor programs to reduce isolation.[38]

Finally, comprehensive care at home can reduce Medicare costs.[39,42] It appears that these improved outcomes are best achieved by multidimensional assessments with at least 9 follow-up home visits. In the second year of the GRACE trial, emergency department and hospital use were significantly reduced.[31]

As transitions of care become more prevalent with today's health care structure, frail elderly patients are at risk of adverse events from errors in information transfer and inability to address rapidly changing health conditions. House calls can smooth patient transitions home from hospitals, acute rehabilitation, and nursing facilities. One study of post-discharge home follow-up by hospital-based nurse practitioners (NPs) compared with usual care for older patients at risk for poor postdischarge outcomes found markedly reduced hospital readmissions, a longer interval to first readmission, and Medicare cost savings of nearly 50% for health care. The success of home visits stems from the fact that they address not only patients' acute conditions but also the chronic comorbid conditions and social issues that put them at risk for poor outcomes, and from the fact that they coordinate the complex care of these individuals in the context of their homes.[43] Transitional care is further discussed by Boling in an article, elsewhere in this issue.

WHAT HAS INFLUENCED RECENT CHANGES IN HOUSE CALLS ACTIVITY?

As mentioned previously, increased reimbursement almost certainly contributed to the rise in Medicare-billed house calls from 1998 to 2007. This trend also reflects growth of both profit- and not-for-profit house calls practices during this period.[23] Such programs provide much needed primary or acute care to homebound and frail, predominantly elderly patients. The programs vary in structure, size, and operation to meet particular geographic, academic, and strategic missions.

Whereas advances in medical technology once threatened the survival of house calls, in the last decade, new mobile medical technology has facilitated expansion of care in the home. The greater availability of intravenous infusion, point-of-care blood testing, pulse oximeters, feeding pumps, ventilators, and mobile radiology enables providers to diagnose and treat patients for conditions that were previously too complex or acute to address at home. Telehealth, broadly defined as programmed telecommunication using interactive video, telephone, and/or the Internet to guide diagnosis, treatment, or prevention, is gaining wider acceptance and may revolutionize the efficiency and capabilities of house calls medicine. New technology is discussed by Bayne in an article, elsewhere in this issue.

Operation of House Calls Practices

House calls practices function differently from office-based care. Successful practices must have clear goals regarding scope of practice and productivity. Some programs are built solely with primary care providers who accept only frail, elderly patients who need home visits for chronic care, and they do not offer urgent care. Depending on the expertise and interest of providers, house calls practices may focus on "hospital at home" models as discussed by Leff and colleagues,[8] assisted living or group home settings, one-time assessments done on request from another provider, terminal care, or patients with behavioral or psychiatric disturbances. Some programs work with other organizations or insurers to provide urgent or transitional care for patients recently discharged from the hospital or identified to be at high risk for rehospitalization. The scope of service dictates professional staffing and the amount and type of organizational infrastructure, including office staff, triage, and portable technology. Excellent communication systems are universally essential.

The types of patients served will dictate where referrals are sought and what type of acute care response capacity is needed. For example, a program designed for primary care to chronically ill patients may target local geriatric practices, home health agencies, and assisted living facilities. If an urgent-care service component is planned, providers need 24-hour phone availability and the capability to make visits on short notice with diagnostic tools. A program focused on palliative care might partner with local hospices and hospital palliative care programs. If the house calls program has limited staffing, the providers may contract with the hospice or home health agency for after-hours coverage and support.

Fewer medical home visits can be done in a day compared with the number of patients typically seen in an office. This is due not only to travel but also because these frail patients often have complex comorbidities. Cognitive or language impairment is prevalent, which necessitates interviewing both patients and caregivers. The average home visit provider sees about 5 patients in a half-day session; office-based practices see about twice that number. For this reason, many nascent house call programs maintain an office-based practice and reserve 1 to 2 sessions per week for home visits until the house calls portion of the practice grows and can stand alone.

Larger programs have hired drivers so that physicians are more efficient during unreimbursed travel time (ordering laboratory work and equipment, charting, and returning phone calls). Academic programs use car time as "teaching" time, giving trainees feedback on physical examination or interviewing skills or discussing how the home setting affects medical management. Much like in office-based practice, this "teaching" time often reduces the number of patients that can be seen in a session.

House calls programs seek to schedule visits in a concentrated geographic zone on a given day, to minimize travel time. In both urban and rural settings, travel is usually done by automobile; however, some providers walk or use public transportation, taxis, or bicycles. The old-fashioned "black bag" is increasingly replaced by a modern house call bag (see **Table 2**). Many urban programs have safety policies, such as making house calls in the morning, having an escort (the "buddy system"), and notifying office staff where providers are working during the day.

Medical documentation and record keeping pose unique challenges. Paper charts should be locked in a separate area of the car or carried by the provider. Many programs now use electronic records, accessed through laptops or other mobile devices, to enable providers to complete documentation on the road. Electronic medical records maintain patient confidentiality, reduce paperwork and threat of loss, and provide continuity when multiple team members within a practice provide care to the same patient. As discussed by Bayne, mobile computing is currently limited by wireless Internet access and slow upload and download speeds.

Private or community-based house calls programs vary in size from just a few patients seen on house calls as part of an office-based practice to large, for-profit multistate groups, some of which provide their own diagnostic testing, which contributes to fiscal margins. Hospital-based house calls programs tend to be larger, multidisciplinary, and partly funded by academic centers due to the large role these programs play in trainee education.[26] There are economic reasons for hospital systems to

Table 2	
Equipment and supplies for the house call bag	
Supplies & Equipment	**Forms & Documents**
Stethoscope	*Letter of introduction to House Call program, including:*
Blood pressure cuff with interchangeable gauge and cuff (regular adult, obese, pediatric)	a. main names and contact numbers of key staff
Gloves (nonsterile and sterile)	b. policies for regular and acute visits
Hemoccult slides & lubricant	c. affiliations with hospitals or other providers, hospices, assisted living or domiciliaries
Otoscope/ophthalmoscope	d. telephone and after-hours availability
Glucometer	e. charges for services
Peak flow meter	
Digital thermometer with disposable probes	*Forms and assessments*
Tape measure	Medical, family, social history
Reflex hammer & tuning fork	Medication review
Sterile 4 × 4 gauze and tape	Physical examination
Toenail clippers	Nutritional assessments
Portable scale	Pain/symptom assessment
Disposable sterile scalpel, forceps, scissors	Functional assessments
Felt tip marking pen	Cognitive screens/assessments
Needles and syringes for aspiration and/or injection	Health care proxy/advance directives
Blood draw supplies	Out of hospital DNR/POLST
Portable sharps container	
Foley catheter and supplies	
Optional	
Fingertip pulse oximeter	
Point of care testing (eg, I-Stat)	
Portable ECG machine	

Abbreviations: DNR, Do not resuscitate; ECG, electrocardiogram; POLST, physician orders for life-sustaining treatment.

Data from American Academy of Home Care Physicians. Making house calls a part of your practice. Edgewood, MD; AAHCP, 2006.

support house calls programs: (1) contribution to hospital revenue via house call patients' hospital admissions; (2) house call provider participation in transitional care for high-risk patients; (3) referrals to hospital-based outpatient specialty services; and (4) potential for philanthropy and positive public relations.[44,45] Some practices are responding to reduced home visit reimbursement by adding nursing home or domiciliary care. Others are filing for nonprofit status, allowing them to raise funds and use philanthropy to cover costs. Concierge practice is also gaining momentum, where physicians opt out of Medicare and charge patients directly for all services, usually in addition to an annual membership fee.

Because of increasing pressure for accountability and value purchasing, providers who bill Medicare, Medicaid, or other commercial insurance should document the need for the medical service to take place at home (medical necessity). However, medical providers are not held to the same definition of homebound status that applies to Medicare home health agencies, which must adhere to an operational definition of "homebound," which defines these patients as those for whom leaving the home is done with difficulty infrequently and is a hardship for the patients and involved caregivers.

WORKING WITH NURSE PRACTITIONERS, PHYSICIAN ASSISTANTS, AND HOME HEALTH AGENCIES

A core concept in geriatric care is the importance of the interdisciplinary team, where each member plays a vital role in the care of the patient. Care in the home especially relies on this model. When a physician stands in a home where there is inadequate food, heat, or needed physical support, these basic needs must be met before a medical care plan has any chance of success. When patients need daily care from nurses and others, a team is essential.

A house calls program must, therefore, identify and develop a team that usually includes partners outside the house call practice itself. In a small private practice, the team may consist of a physician, who sees patients in the office 3 days per week and does home visits the other 2 days, a community nursing agency, and the office nurse who answers urgent calls, handles medication refills, and helps with paperwork (approval of services) associated with home medical care. In a larger house call program, a team may consist of several physicians, NPs and physician assistants (PAs) providing routine and urgent home visits, registered nurses, social workers, and support staff. Collaboration of multiple disciplines provides needed services to a patient with the goal of providing comprehensive home-based care and preventing hospitalizations. To cultivate teamwork when providers are dispersed, regular team meetings are important for team building and identifying key medical and social issues.

Many practices include NPs or PAs as physician extenders. Some NPs and PAs work in collaboration with physicians, co-managing patient panels, while others work independently with physician oversight and support. Each state has its own rules regarding licensure and supervision. Medicare recognizes NPs as providers who can treat patients and order tests but reimburses at 85% of the physician rate. Medicare skilled home care orders must be signed by the physician as a matter of federal statute.

Most house calls practices have strong relationships with other community services, including home health care and hospice agencies, volunteer organizations, meals-on-wheels programs, senior case managers, and Adult Protective Services. These collaborations enable delivery of comprehensive medical and psychosocial care plans, and communication is vital to success.

House calls practices are organized in a variety of ways, which generally fall under two broad categories as described below.

- Clinic-based practice: Physicians make home visits before or after work or at designated times during the week. Some practices have NPs or PAs who make visits, either for acute issues or chronic follow-up care. Benefits of this model include that patients can move in and out of clinic as their health status changes. Challenges include responding to acute care needs at home when providers are seeing scheduled patients in clinic and limiting the geography that can be covered.
- Mobile practice: Physicians make home visits full time or partner with NPs or PAs to provide daily visits. Some offer evening or weekend care. Some physicians

incorporate medical assistants as drivers and assistants during visits. Others keep medical assistants in the office to triage phone calls and paperwork. Benefits include reduced overhead and flexible schedules. Challenges include lack of clinic support and infrastructure, which can be overcome by team communication and information technology.

REGIONAL VARIATION IN MARKET PENETRATION

Communities including San Diego, Miami, Phoenix, New York, and Detroit have larger organizations that provide substantial numbers of home visits (several thousand per month). Relatively large home medical care companies that employ dozens of physicians exist in some regions of the country. Some of these organizations partner with insurers to target chronically ill and elderly patients who pose high risk for the insurance plan and provide home visits in conjunction with regular primary care visits to prevent emergency room visits and costly hospitalizations. In other areas, only a few physicians provide this service, and unmet need abounds.

CARE QUALITY AND CERTIFICATION FOR HOME MEDICAL CARE PROVIDERS

As has been true with other emerging fields of medical practice, home medical care does not yet have national standards. The American Academy of Home Care Physicians has developed a code of ethics, educational programs, and a certification examination, which may become the basis for standardization as the field grows. A nationally representative group of home care providers also derived a set of quality indicators for home medical care based on the validated Assessing Care of Vulnerable Elders guidelines.[46] For reasons of cost, most practices are not accredited by organizations that evaluate quality of care, such as the Joint Commission; accredited house call programs are usually affiliated with hospitals and health systems. There are accepted general standards for provider certification, such as primary specialty boards, and subspecialty qualification, such as geriatrics. Board certification in palliative care emerged in 1996 under the American Board of Hospice and Palliative Medicine and was finally recognized by the American Board of Medical Subspecialties in 2008. However, the unique knowledge specific to home health care practice is not really tested or addressed by these other organizations and is an area in need of further attention as this type of care becomes more prevalent in the nation.

REFERENCES

1. Starr P. The social transformation of American medicine. New York: Basic Books; 1982. p. 359.
2. Driscoll CE. Is there a doctor in the house? Am Acad Home Care Physicians News 1991;3:7–8.
3. Cherry DK, Burt CW, Woodwell DA. National ambulatory medical care survey: 2001 summary. Adv data 2003;11:337.
4. Meyer GS, Gibbons RV. House calls to the elderly—a vanishing practice among physicians. N Engl J Med 1997;337:1815–20.
5. Aylin P, Majeed FA, Cook DG, et al. Home visiting by general practitioners in England and Wales. BMJ 1996;313:207–10.
6. Keenan JM, Hepburn KW. The role of physicians in home health care. Clin Geriatr Med 1991;7:665–75.
7. Elkan R, Kendrick D, Dewey M, et al. Effectiveness of home based support for older people: systematic review and meta-analysis. BMJ 2001;323:1–9.

8. Leff B, Burton JR. Acute medical care in the home. J Am Geriatr Soc 1996;44: 603–5.
9. Berenson A, Abelson R. Weighing the costs of a CT scan's look inside the heart. New York Times June 29, 2008.
10. McArthur WJ. Geriatric house calls: relic of the past or challenge of the future? Can Fam Physician 1990;36:1409–11, 1415.
11. Boling PA, Retchin SM, Ellis J, et al. Factors associated with the frequency of house calls by primary care physicians. J Gen Intern Med 1991;6:335–40.
12. Taler G. House calls for the 21st century. J Am Geriatr Soc 1998;46:246–8.
13. Haupt B, Hing E, Strahan G. The national home and hospice care survey: 1992. [summary]. Vital Health Stat 1 1994;117:1–110.
14. Office of Inspector General, DHHS 1997. Operation restore trust: audit of Medicare home health services in California, Illinois, A-04-96-02121. Office of the Inspector General Press Office.
15. Muramatsu N, Cornwell T. Needs of physician house calls—views from health and social service providers. Home Health Care Serv Q 2003;22:17–29.
16. Moore G, Showstack J. Primary care medicine in crisis: toward reconstruction and renewal. Ann Intern Med 2003;138:244–7.
17. Colwill JM, Cultice JM, Kruse RL. Will generalist physician supply meet demands of an increasing and aging population? Health Aff 2008;27:w232–41.
18. ADGAP. Status of Geriatrics Workforce Study. Available at: http://www. adgapstudy.uc.edu/FAQ.cfm. Accessed July 20, 2008.
19. Steel RK, Musliner M, Boling PA. Medical schools and home care. NEJM 1994; 331:1098–9.
20. Committee on the Future Health Care Workforce for Older Americans, Institute of Medicine. Retooling for an aging America: building the health care workforce. Washington (DC): The National Academies Press; 2008.
21. Administration on Aging, US Department of Health and Human Services. A profile of older Americans: Washington (DC); Administration of Aging, US Department of Health and Human Services. 2007.
22. Boling PA. The physician's role in home health care. Caring 1998;17:10–5.
23. Leff B, Burton JR. The future history of home care and physician house calls in the United States. J Gerontol 2001;56A:M603–8.
24. Direct data source: Medicare Part B Summary Data 2005–2007; file prepared for American Academy of Home Care Physicians, August 2008.
25. Landers SH, Gunn PW, Flocke SA, et al. Trends in house calls to Medicare beneficiaries. JAMA 2005;294:2435–6.
26. Smith KL, Ornstein K, Soriano T, et al. A multidisciplinary program for delivering primary care to the underserved urban homebound: looking back, moving forward. J Am Geriatr Soc 2006;54:1283–9.
27. Available at: http://www.aahcp.org/presentations2008/boling_billing_coding_update_boling.ppt. Accessed September 22, 2008.
28. Available at: http://www.aahcp.org/medicare_paymenthistory_2004-2010.pdf. Accessed October 2, 2008.
29. AGS. Role of house calls in geriatric practice—clinical practice statement. Available at: www.americangeriatrics.org/products/positionpapers/housecallPF.shtml. Accessed April 18, 2008.
30. Reuben DB, Fried TR, Wachtel TJ, et al. When the patient cannot come to the doctor: a medical house calls program. J Am Geriatr Soc 1998;46:226–31.
31. Counsell SR, Callahan CM, Clark DO, et al. Geriatric care management for low-income seniors: a randomized controlled trial. JAMA 2007;298:2623–33.

32. Yuen JK, Breckman R, Adelman RD, et al. Reflections of medical students on visiting chronically ill older patients in the home. J Am Geriatr Soc 2006;54: 1778–83.
33. Stuck AE, Minder CE, Peter-Wuest I, et al. A randomized trial of in-home visits for disability prevention in community-dwelling older people at low and high risk for nursing home admission. Arch Intern Med 2000;160:977–86.
34. Ramsdell JW, Swart JO, Jackson JE, et al. The yield of a home visit in the assessment of geriatric patients. J Am Geriatr Soc 1989;37:17–24.
35. Ramsdell JW, Jackson JE, Guy JH, et al. Comparison of clinic-based home assessment to a home visit in demented elderly patients. Alzheimer Dis Assoc Disord 2004;18:145–53.
36. Brumley RD, Enguidanos S, Cherin DA. Effectiveness of a home-based palliative care program for end-of-life. J Palliat Med 2003;6:715–24.
37. Ciemins EL, Stuart B, Gerber R, et al. An evaluation of the advanced illness management (AIM) program: increasing hospice utilization in the San Francisco Bay area. J Palliat Med 2006;9:1404–11.
38. Stuck AE, Aranow HU, Steiner A, et al. A trial of annual in-home comprehensive geriatric assessments for elderly people living in the community. NEJM 1995;333: 1184–9.
39. Yudin J, Kinosian B, Graub PB, et al [ElderPAC]. Available at: www.aahcp.org/ presentations; 2005; Accessed June 23, 2008.
40. Stuck AE, Egger M, Hammer A, et al. Home visits to prevent nursing home admission and functional decline in elderly people. JAMA 2002;287:1022–8.
41. Gurley RJ, Lum N, Sande M, et al. Persons found in their home helpless or dead. NEJM 1996;334:1710–6.
42. Phillips S. Home based chronic care. Available at: www.aahcp.org/presentations/ 2005. Accessed June 23, 2008.
43. Naylor MD, Brooten D, Campbell R, et al. Comprehensive discharge planning and home follow-up of hospitalized elders. JAMA 1999;281:613–20.
44. Desai NR, Smith KL, Boal J. The positive financial contribution of home-based primary care programs: the case of the Mount Sinai visiting doctors. J Am Geriatr Soc 2008;56:744–9.
45. Smigelski C, Hungate B, Holdren J, et al. Transitional model of care at VCU medical center—6 years' experience. AGS Annual Meeting Abstract April 2008.
46. Smith KL, Soriano TA, Boal J. Brief communication: national quality-of-care standards in home-based primary care. Ann Intern Med 2007;146:188–92.

Advances and Issues in Personal Care

Robyn Stone, DrPH[a], Robert Newcomer, PhD[b],*

KEYWORDS

- Personal assistant services • Home care • Long term care
- Community based care

People of all ages with disabilities may need help from other people in performing activities of daily living (ADL), such as bathing, dressing, bladder and bowel management, and eating and instrumental activities of daily living (IADL), such as shopping for groceries, preparing meals, managing finances, and taking medications. Such help is often termed *personal assistance services* (PAS). PAS is generally classified into (1) informal (unpaid) services provided by family members, friends and neighbors and (2) formal services that are paid for directly out of pocket or by public payers, private insurance, or other sources.

PAS is available in both community and non-community settings (like nursing homes) and known under various job titles. Among these are direct service workers; home care aides or workers; homemaker/chore workers; and personal care aides, workers, or attendants. The focus of this article is on paid workers in community settings. Community-based PAS is considered to be "nonskilled" assistance. It usually does not require supervision by health professionals or other licensed providers, although many paid workers are employed by agencies that may be licensed. An emergent approach in PAS is for clients to self-direct their care and for workers to be independent providers employed directly by the care recipient.

The number of persons involved as either a PAS recipient or provider is large and growing. Nationally, more than 5.4 million community-dwelling adults have limitations in at least 1 ADL, and about 3 times this number have limitations in IADLs.[1] Projections indicate that the number of people needing help in ADLs or IADLs will more than double, going to 27 million in 2050.[2] Commensurate with the growth in need has been a growth in the number of paid PAS workers. Estimates derived from the American Community Survey show that the number of providers increased from about a quarter of a million in 1989 to more than a million in 2005.[3] This growth in home and

This article was prepared with the support of funding from the National Institute on Disability and Rehabilitation Research (#H133B031008) and the Centers for Disease Control (#200-2007-207).
[a] Institute for the Future of Aging Services, Washington, DC, USA
[b] Center for Personal Assistance Services, University of California, San Francisco, USA
* Corresponding author.
E-mail address: robert.newcomer@ucsf.edu (R. Newcomer).

Clin Geriatr Med 25 (2009) 35–45
doi:10.1016/j.cger.2008.10.004
0749-0690/08/$ – see front matter

community-based care occurred in both public and privately paid programs and afforded the opportunity for many individuals who might otherwise be in nursing homes or housing with services to remain in the community. Public concerns about cost, access, and the adequacy of assistance have paralleled this growth.

WHO ARE THE RECIPIENTS?

More than 80% of PAS hours are provided by unpaid, informal caregivers, such as family members. However, a recent analysis, using the 1994–1997 National Health Interview Survey on Disability, found that of the 13.2 million American adults receiving some form of PAS, almost 25% (3.2 million) received some help from 1 or more paid workers. Further, this analysis estimated that people living in the community receiving help in 1 or more ADL received an average of 57 hours of help per week.[4] A larger population (about 8.3 million people) who received help with 1 or more IADL, but no ADLs, got an average of 16 hours of help per week. The same study found that individuals with unmet need for personal assistance have a shortfall of 13 hours of help per week compared with those with met need. Unmet need is defined by the extent to which needed assistance is unavailable or insufficient. The shortfall in hours was much greater among persons who lived alone than that among those who lived with others (22 versus 10 hours). Rates of unmet need increased as the number of ADL limitations and chronic health conditions increased and among black or Hispanic individuals, among those in apartments, and when there was limited insurance coverage. Living with a spouse and use of equipment and assistive devices were associated with reduced unmet need. Overall, less than 6% of needed hours are unmet among the 3.3 million people needing help in 2 or more ADLs.

Unmet need for PAS is an important policy issue. People who do not get the help they need are at risk of institutionalization and are far more likely than those getting adequate help to experience adverse consequences, including discomfort, weight loss, dehydration, falls, burns, and dissatisfaction with the amount of help received.[5] Rates of acute hospital admissions have been shown to be higher for people whose needs are unmet than for those with met needs.[6]

PAS WORKFORCE

The availability of paid PAS is of great benefit to people needing services that supplement or replace that available from informal providers. More than one million persons are estimated to be employed as PAS workers in community settings.[3] There are also an estimated 1.4 million direct care workers (eg, nurses' aides, home health aides, and personal care aides) working in nursing homes, personal care facilities, home care agencies, residential care, or other organizations (eg, hospitals and rehabilitation centers) providing assistance with ADLs and IADLs for persons with disability and the aged.[7,8]

Most of what is known about the PAS workforce comes from studies of public program participants and their providers. Within this limitation, between 80% and 90% of direct care workers are women. The typical worker is a single mother between age 25 and 54 years.[9] PAS workers are ethnically diverse. One in five workers is foreign born, and many are educated in another country.[10] One-third are African American and 15% are either non-white Hispanics or other workers of color.[11]

Concerns about the adequacy of and access to PAS in the future in some measure are based on concern about labor supply. In 2000, the ratio of women aged 20 to 54 years to persons aged 85+ years was 16:1. By 2010, the ratio will drop to about 12:1. These ratios are estimated to fall to 8.5:1 and 5.7:1 by 2030 and 2040, respectively.[9]

Recognizing that the aged are but 1 source of demand for personal care assistance, it is apparent that the workforce supply will become increasingly problematic if PAS retention problems are not resolved or if a new labor source is not identified. This affects both formal or paid direct care paraprofessionals and family caregivers.

The availability of workers is far from uniform. This is illustrated by an analysis that compared the number of PAS workers in each state divided by the number of people with ADL difficulties in that state. The result ranged widely (eg, 49 workers per 1,000 people in Mississippi to 269 in New York).[12,13] This disparity was partly due to differences in Medicaid spending on noninstitutional long-term services and to differences in the availability of workers to fill the demand. Access to formal PAS has been found to be a particular problem for people living in rural areas and the South, other than North Carolina.

A number of additional factors contribute to the undersupply of direct care PAS workers, particularly wages and benefits. Median hourly wages in 2006 ranged from $6.41 (in Texas) to $13.64 (in Alaska) or $8.54 nationally. This is an annual wage of between $13,333 and $28,371, assuming the worker works full time. Many service workers are employed much less than full time. Since 2000, adjusting for inflation, real wages for PAS workers has declined by 4% nationally. Even in the 29 states showing an increase in real annual median wages over this 7-year period, only 5 had an annual median wage increase of 2% or more.[14] The evaluation of the national Cash & Counseling Demonstration, which enabled disabled beneficiaries to hire and fire their PAS workers and pay them directly, found that wages of consumer-directed workers were about 15% higher than those of agency-directed workers in 2 of the 3 demonstration states but 5% less in the other state.[15]

Not surprisingly, almost 30% of direct care paraprofessionals live in poverty and are more likely than many workers to rely on public benefits to supplement their wages.[16] Among single-parent workers, 30% to 35% receive food stamps. A similar proportion of workers also rely on publicly funded health care.[9] Even those working for provider organizations (as opposed to those who are self-employed) have limited access to benefits. For example, 40% of home health aides have *no* health insurance, and 75% have *no* employer sponsored-pensions.[17] Access to insurance and other benefits is thought to be even lower among self-employed and family caregiver aides.

There are limited requirements and skills needed to become a PAS worker. The position does not require high-school education or English proficiency. Formal training, if required, is minimal (eg, up to 75 hours if working in a Medicare- or Medicaid-certified organization, and less if with other employers).[18] These limited requirements place PAS in competition with entry-level jobs in other service industry sectors of the economy (eg, fast food) that pay comparable or higher hourly wages, offer more certainty with respect to work schedules and full-time salaries, and even such minimal benefits as sick days, holidays, and health insurance.[8,9] For PAS workers who are independent providers, especially those employed by private pay clients, training other than that given by the client and family may be minimal.[19] Additionally, when family members are the paid providers, as is the case in many consumer-directed programs, there may be resistance to obtaining training.

Further complicating matters are that PAS and PAS-related positions are often physically and emotionally demanding, with few opportunities for advancement in the same work role and often accompanied by worker perceptions that their jobs lack respect from supervisors and care recipients. A recent national report on the mental health status associated with various occupations noted that 11% of PAS workers reported being depressed for two or more weeks, the highest rate of depression experience observed in any of the 21 occupational categories that were tracked.[20] Also, limited job training and supervision are thought to contribute to injuries and illness in this workforce.

Occupational injury among home-based care workers is known in other countries to be a prevalent problem.[21,22] Injury data in the United States (such as those from the Bureau of Labor Statistics [BLS]) generally do not differentiate between community-based and institution-based workers. Moreover, these data come almost exclusively from agencies, ignoring independent providers. Nevertheless, the 2003 BLS survey provides illustrative injury-rate data.[23,24] It reported that the injury rate in nursing homes and residential homes was 10.1 per 100 full-time equivalents FTEs for all employees. This rate is double that of the all industry rate of 5.0 per 100 FTEs.[23]

An extrapolation of these injury rates into community settings, after adjusting for comparable levels of need among the PAS recipients, would likely produce an underestimate of worker injuries. Hospital and nursing home workers are generally thought to have more training, experience, supervision, and access to supplemental assistance as necessary compared with home care providers. Studies of home health care workers, a related occupation, support the hypothesis about differential risk. For example, Myers and colleagues[25] found higher injury rates among home health workers than those among hospital and nursing home workers. The annual rate of low-back injuries among home health workers was 15.4 per 100 FTEs compared with 5.9 per 100 FTEs for hospital nursing aides. A survey of 1900 home care workers in Washington state found that almost 40% of the respondents had experienced a work-related injury or health problem (including muscle strain and emotional stress); 26% reported experiencing discrimination, harassment, or abuse (especially verbal) on the job.[26]

In combination, the working situation, injuries, and low wages and benefits contribute to a high rate of annual staff turnover. This rate is 40% to 60% among direct service workers generally.[27] Further, many programs report that a third or more of persons who undertake training either never take positions or leave positions within the first 3 months. These rates suggest problems in recruitment and screening of position applicants as well as perhaps the training itself. The high rate of turnover of staff once on the job is problematic for quality and continuity of care as well. Among other things, turnover is a burden for clients who must continually gain confidence in their care provider. It is also a financial and psychological burden on organizations (and families hiring independent providers) that incur significant replacement costs and payers who must continually provide training; and it is a burden on coworkers who must absorb the increased workload.[28] For disabled persons receiving care at home, the need to continually train new workers for the specific care required and the anxiety over whether workers show up for work or stay on the job for even a short period of time is stressful and time-consuming.[29]

WHO PAYS?

A number of government programs support PAS in the United States, including Medicaid, Title XX Social Security block grants, Title III Older Americans Act funds, state (and local government) general funds, and the Department of Veterans Affairs Aids and Attendance Program. The Medicare home health benefit offers some unskilled assistance as well but usually on a short-term and very limited basis after hospitalization. The federal government spent an estimated $40 billion on PAS for people living at home and about $104 billion for institutional care in 2002.[30] Private financing, though not well documented or studied, is thought to be prevalent. This occurs most commonly through out-of-pocket payments, but long-term care insurance also covers this benefit.

Medicaid is, by far, the most significant of the public programs for PAS. Historically, home and community-based service (HCBS) alternatives have been an optional benefit within Medicaid. Since 1975, the US Congress and state legislatures have steadily expanded funding for HCBS through two main programs: PAS Optional State Benefit and HCBS waivers. The 1999 Supreme Court decision in Olmstead v. L.C., 119 S. Ct. 2176 provided a legal precedent requiring states to offer persons with disabilities appropriate alternatives to institutional placement when (1) professionals reasonably determine that such placement is appropriate and (2) the placement can be reasonably accommodated. This ruling, based on the Americans with Disabilities Act (initially adopted in 1990), entitles people with disabilities the right to live in the most integrated setting, but it raises numerous questions about what states must do to ensure access to choices between institutional placements and HCBS.

Personal care services can be included (but are not mandatory) in the Medicaid benefit package. Medicaid PAS programs typically provide services through home care or personal attendant agencies, but some states (most notably, California with more than 400,000 recipients) predominantly use independent providers selected, managed, and dismissed by the Medicaid participants. Thirty states reported an active PAS optional state plan benefit in 2002 (up from 26 in 1999) and that 45 states offered some PAS through at least one HCBS waiver.[31]

The Medicaid HCBS waiver program was established with the passage of Section 2176 of the Omnibus Budget Reconciliation Act of 1981. Unlike the Optional Personal Care program, waiver regulations require HCBS waiver services to be limited to those who are eligible for institutional placement. Further, states are allowed to target waivers to particular populations, so they are not required to offer waiver services to all categorically or medically needy groups, and they may limit the number of individuals who may receive benefits. Waivers can be used to serve a broad range of populations, including the aged and younger physically disabled, individuals with developmental disabilities, and others with a variety of conditions and chronic disorders, such as acquired immunodeficiency syndrome (AIDS), acquired brain injuries, and other forms of severe disability, including, to a limited extent, chronic mental illness. In addition to PAS services, these programs can offer case management, homemaker/chore services, adult day care, and transportation to waiver-eligible individuals.

While PAS programs are growing, the majority of Medicaid dollars still pay for institutional care (primarily for elderly nursing home residents). Only seven states spent 40% or more of their Medicaid long-term care dollars on PAS programs. There is great state variation, furthermore, in the proportion of Medicaid long-term care spending going toward PAS, ranging from 1% in Tennessee to 55% in Oregon.[32]

PROGRAM INNOVATIONS

Since 2002, Centers for Medicare and Medicaid Services (CMS) has introduced several programs to further facilitate state PAS development. This activity, often referred to as "balancing," is intended to increase the number of people with PAS needs served in their homes or in more home-like settings in their communities and decrease the number in nursing homes. The effect is to shift more resources toward PAS, to "balance" Medicaid long-term care spending between institutional services and HCBS.[32] One of the most visible efforts is the CMS New Freedom Initiative (2002). It is designed to increase access to assistive technologies, expand educational opportunities, increase integration into the workforce, and promote increased access to daily community life. Another major program is the Money Follows the Person initiative

(2007). It seeks to accelerate the development of programs that facilitate the transition from nursing homes to home and community-based settings.

Another major innovation in the past decade has been the expansion of consumer-directed options within PAS programs. Four out of five states offer consumer-directed options for PAS, although this is usually a small component of their PAS delivery system.[33,34] This approach empowers the consumer to make critical decisions about hiring and firing workers and to manage one's own services to meet individual needs and preferences. States offer the elements of consumer-directed care either through independent providers or agency arrangements that permit the recipient some control over the choice and supervision of the PAS worker. Registries, fiscal intermediaries, and other organizations have been developed to facilitate the match of consumers and providers for the delivery of PAS through independent providers, but the quality of this support is variable within and between states.[19]

The most distinctive example of consumer direction is the Cash & Counseling Demonstration. This demonstration and its evaluation were supported by the Robert Wood Johnson Foundation and the US Department of Health and Human Services to test the feasibility and efficacy of allowing Medicaid waiver enrollees in Arkansas, Florida, and New Jersey to hire and fire their own workers, including paying family members. Participating states give the recipient a voucher payment to purchase needed assistance; some limit the expenditures to a specified array of services. The evaluation outcomes have, for the most part, been positive, and they support findings from other studies of consumer direction that this approach allows individuals with disabilities across the age span greater freedom and control over the direction of their own personal care choices. Improved patient satisfaction, increased community involvement, and reduced unmet needs have also been seen. At least 12 other states have pursued this strategy through the waiver authority.

Some concerns have been raised about paying family members in consumer-directed programs. An evaluation of the In Home Supportive Services Program (IHSS)—California's Medicaid-funded PAS program—found that parents paid as providers for minor children and spouses paid as caregivers tended to have recipients with comparable or higher service needs relative to recipients with nonrelatives or other relatives paid as providers. Further, after adjusting for health conditions and functional limitations, average monthly Medicaid expenditures and nursing home use were lower among those with legally responsible relatives.[35]

EXPANDING AND STRENGTHENING THE PAS WORKFORCE

A number of current and future trends are converging to highlight the need for federal, state, and private sector efforts to strengthen and expand the PAS workforce. These include aging of the population, extended longevity across all groups of people with disabilities, changing needs of unpaid caregivers who are susceptible to burnout, and increasing lack of the traditional labor pool of women aged 35 to 54 years who are most likely to hold PAS jobs. There are a number of ways in which the federal and state governments, along with the private sector, can begin to solve the short- and long-term workforce challenges.

Expand the PAS Workforce

Throwing warm bodies at the long-term care problem will not solve the vexing financing and quality problems that are at the heart of the need to reform long-term care. However, most stakeholders would agree that new sources of caregivers must be attracted to meet future demand for PAS workers. The federal and state governments, first of all, must do a better job of tracking supply and demand and labor shortage areas. Employers, consumers, labor unions, and state policy makers should collaborate to develop and launch marketing and recruiting campaigns aimed at modernizing the image of long-term care as a career choice. Federal and state funders and employers also need to understand the extent to which lack of resources to pay for training is a barrier to recruitment and to assist where financial help is needed. The connection between government-supported workforce investment activities, totaling more than $5 billion in 2005, and the needs of long-term care employers and consumers for qualified PAS workers should be strengthened. National, state, and municipal efforts need to be launched to channel more of these resources to the recruitment and training of the long-term care workforce.

Create Competitive Jobs Through Wage and Benefit Enhancements

Almost all stakeholders agree that low wages for PAS workers and limited employer-based health insurance coverage make recruiting and retaining personnel in the long-term care industry difficult. In the long term, improving wages and benefits for long-term care personnel is tied to fundamental reforms in how long-term care is financed and reimbursed. In the shorter term, states and providers, working in partnership with federal funders, should examine strategies for raising wages and providing health insurance to this workforce, including implementing "pay for performance" schemes and improving the impact of "Medicaid wage pass-through," a policy that increases Medicaid reimbursement to providers, with the expectation that such an increase will be directly passed through to personnel in the form of higher wages or benefits. Additional strategies to increase PAS worker compensation and benefits include collective bargaining, minimum wage improvements, health insurance initiatives and additional benefits, transportation subsidies, and the development of career ladders.[36]

Improve Working Conditions and the Quality of the PAS Job

Higher wages and better benefits will not be sufficient in and of themselves to attract a high-quality workforce. Most experts agree that working conditions and the quality of the job must be improved. Efforts should include the development of effective managers and management practices in PAS agencies, increasing participation of racial and ethnic minorities in PAS management, developing financial incentives and regulatory relief for states and employers that have achieved real progress in improving working conditions while maintaining high standards of quality, promoting self-assessment and reporting of working conditions in agency-based and consumer-directed programs, and developing career advancement pathways for PAS workers.

Job Training

A clear link has yet to be established between increased training and increased recruitment and retention but there is general consensus that quality training will help to sustain a viable paid and unpaid PAS workforce and lead to higher quality of assistance. Training has been required for paid PAS workers in nursing homes, assisted living, and home health and other Medicaid- or Medicare-certified agencies, but training is not required (and is consequently limited) for most PAS community-based workers in most states. Training needs for both paid and unpaid PAS workers in community settings seem to be increasing, especially for individuals providing informal medical tasks and day-to-day care.[13,37] Further, a recent study suggests that the strategies employed by regulators and educators to prepare the workforce and to assure that the caregivers are able to keep pace with changes in the technical knowledge base and new technologies are not effective. Further, there is a huge shortfall of personnel who are competent and committed to educating and preparing PAS workers for their jobs.[13]

Training for PAS workers in the United States is at a very rudimentary stage of development. This is true for three reasons: (1) no federal *requirements* exist related to PAS worker training, and state requirements vary widely and, generally, are weak and inconsistent; (2) PAS worker training *curricula* are often mediocre; and (3) few states have taken steps to create, fund, or otherwise support PAS training *infrastructure*, which supports training for PAS workers. A report that examined state requirements for Medicaid-funded personal care services found 301 sets of requirements for PAS across Medicaid programs in all 50 states and the District of Columbia.[38] The median number of required training hours was only 28, but nearly half of the requirements did not specify the required training hours. Furthermore, 26% of training requirements allowed attendants to begin work before completing the required training.

On a positive note, Centers for Independent Living and many state Medicaid programs have recently been implementing training programs for community-based caregivers and the consumer-directed PAS workforce. Additionally, 11 states are developing innovative approaches, such as establishing career ladders and training opportunities for PAS workers, and 5 are considering these types of opportunities.[39,40] Further, a number of states (eg, Michigan, Pennsylvania, Oregon, and Washington) are exploring the development of competency-based curricula for PAS training.[41,42] Most of these efforts are designed to establish a set of core standards and training programs for PAS workers across the continuum of services and community-based settings.

There is a need to make education and training opportunities more accessible, particularly in rural areas. Incentives could be provided to community colleges and other educational vendors to broaden participation in formal instruction for PAS workers. Techniques such as satellite broadcasts, Web-based courses, flexible scheduling of courses, easily accessible locations, and on-the-job training opportunities, such as the Department of Labor apprenticeship models, should be pursued.

Expanding the Scope of Practice

Finally, one of the major regulatory barriers that greatly affects the ability of PAS workers to effectively do their job and obtain advancement opportunities is being contested. This is the extent of nurse delegation allowed for PAS workers in each state. Generally, direct care workers are restricted from performing certain tasks such as medication management and caring for wounds. Several states have modified the nurse delegation provision to varying degrees to allow home care aides in assisted living and home-based settings to engage in these tasks. Nine states have specific consumer-directed care exemptions in their nurse practice regulations that allow independent providers to have a broader scope of practice.[43] The use of legally responsible relatives as PAS providers is another means to broaden the scope of practice, as spouses and parents would be allowed to perform functions such as medication management. These expanded tasks are often not accompanied by requiring training of family providers, nor have the outcomes of these approaches been formally evaluated.

REFERENCES

1. National Center for Health Statistics. 1994 National health interview survey on disability, phase I and II: CD-ROM Series 10, number 8a. Hyattsville (MD): U.S. Department of Health and Human Services, Centers for Disease Control; 1998.

2. US Department of Health and Human Services. The future supply of long-term care workers in relation to the aging baby boom generation: report to congress. Washington, DC: Department of Health & Human Services; 2003.
3. Kaye HS, Chapman S, Newcomer R, et al. The personal assistance workforce: trends in supply and demand. Health Aff 2006;25(4):1113–20.
4. LaPlante MP, Harrington C, Kang T. Estimating paid and unpaid hours of personal assistance services in activities of daily living provided to adults living at home. Health Services Research 2002;37(2):397–415.
5. LaPlante MP, Kaye S, Kang T, et al. Unmet need for personal assistance services: estimating the shortfall in hours of help and adverse consequences. J Gerontol B Psychol Sci Soc Sci 2004;59b(2):S98–108.
6. Sands LP, Wnag Y, McCabe GP, et al. Rates of acute care admissions for frail older people living with met versus unmet activities of daily living needs. J Am Geriatr Soc 2008;54(2):339–44.
7. Bureau of Labor Statistics. Survey of occupational injuries and illnesses, 2003. Washington, DC: US Dept of Labor; 2003. OMB No. 1220-0045. BLS-9300 W06.
8. Center for Health Workforce Studies. The impact of the aging population on the health workforce in the United States. School of Public Health, SUNY Albany. Albany (NY): Center for Health Workforce Studies; 2005.
9. US General Accounting Office (US GAO). Nursing workforce: recruitment and retention of nurses and nurse aides is a growing concern. Testimony before the committee on health, education, labor, and pensions. Washington, DC: US Senate; 2001.
10. Leutz WN. Immigration and the elderly: foreign-born workers in long-term care. Immigration Policy in Focus 2007;5(12):1–12.
11. Montgomery RJ, Holley L, Deichert J, et al. A profile of home care personnel from the 2000 census: how it changes what we know. Gerontologist 2005;45: 593–600.
12. Kaye S. Trends in the PAS workforce. Paper presented at the state of the science conference: meeting the nation's need for personal assistance services. Washington, DC: National Press Club; 2007.
13. Harahan MF, Stone RI. Who Will Care? Building the Geriatric Long-Term Care Labor Force. In: Hudson RB, editor. Boomer Bust? Economic and Political Issues of the Graying Society. Westport (CT): Praeger Publishing; 2008.
14. PHI. State chart book on wages for personal and home care aides, 1999–2006. San Francisco: Center for Personal Assistance Services, University of California; 2008.
15. Dale S, Brown R, Phillips B, et al. The experiences of workers hired under cash and counseling: findings from Arkansas, Florida, and New Jersey. Final report. Princeton, NJ: Mathematica Policy Research; 2005.
16. Case BG, Himmelstein DU, Woolhandler S, et al. No care for the caregivers: declining health insurance coverage for health care personnel & their children 1988–1998. Am J Public Health 2002;92(3):404–8.
17. Crown W, Ahlburg D, MacAdam M, et al. The demographic and employment characteristics of home care aides: a comparison with nursing home aides, hospital aides, and other workers. The Gerontologist 1995;35(2):162–70.
18. Stone RI. Frontline workers in long-term care: a background paper. Washington, DC: American Association of Homes and Services for the Aging; 2001a.
19. Scherzer T, Wong A, Newcomer R. Financial management services in consumer-directed programs. Home Health Care Serv Q 2007;26(1):29–42.

20. Substance Abuse and Mental Health Services Administration. Depression among adults employed full-time, by occupational category. NSDUH Report. Rockville (MD): SAMHSA; 2007.

21. Ono Y, Lagerstrom M, Hagberg M, et al. Reports of work related musculoskeletal injury among home care service workers compared with nursery school workers and the general population of employed women in Sweden. Occup Environ Med 1995;52:686–93.

22. Dellve L, Lagerstrom M, Hagberg M, et al. Work-system risk factors for permanent work disability among home-care workers: a case-control study. Int Arch Occup Environ Health 2003;76:216–24.

23. Bureau of Labor Statistics. Table 1. Incidence rates of nonfatal occupational injuries and illnesses by industry and case types, 2003. Available at: http://www.bls.gov/iif/osh/os/ostb13555.pdf. Accessed on June 12, 2007.

24. Bureau of Labor Statistics. Lost-work time injuries and illnesses: characteristics and resulting days away from work, 2003 (News Release). Washington, DC: US Department of Labor; 2005a.

25. Myers A, Jensen RC, Nestor D, et al. Low back injuries among home health aides compared with hospital nursing aides. Home Health Care Serv Q 1993;14(2/3):149–55.

26. Hayashi R, Gibson JW, Weatherley RA, et al. Working conditions in home care: a survey of Washington state's home care workers. Home Health Care Serv Q 1994;14(4):37–48.

27. Stone RI. Research on workers in long-term care. Generations 2001b;25(1):49–57.

28. Stone RI. Long-term care for the elderly with disabilities: current policy, emerging trends, and implications for the 21st century. New York: Milbank Memorial Fund; 2000.

29. Dale SB, Brown RS. How does Cash & Counseling affect costs? Health Serv Res 2007;42(1, pt.2):488–509.

30. Kitchener M, Ng T, Harrington C, et al. Medicaid home and community-based services: National program trends. Health Aff 2005;24(1):206–12.

31. Kitchener M, Ng T, Harrington C, et al. Medicaid State Plan personal care services: trends in programs and policies. J Health Soc Policy 2007a;19(3):9–26.

32. Kassner E, Reinhard S, Fox-Grage W, et al. A balancing act: state long-term care reform. (Report #2008-10). Washington, DC: AARP Public Policy Institute; 2008.

33. Kitchener M, Ng T, Harrington C, et al. Medicaid home and community-based services for the elderly: trends in programs and policies. J Appl Gerontol 2007b;26(3):303–24.

34. Foster L, Brown R, Phillips B, et al. Improving the quality of Medicaid personal assistance through consumer direction. Health Aff Jan–Jun;Suppl Web Exclusives:W3–162–75. 2003.

35. Newcomer R, Kang T. Analysis of the California in home supportive services (IHSS) plus waiver demonstration program. Final report. Washington, DC: Office of the Assistant Secretary for Planning & Evaluation, Department of Health & Human Services; 2008.

36. Seavey D, Salter V. Paying for quality care: Strategies for improving wages and benefits for personal care assistants. Washington, DC: AARP Public Policy Institute; 2006.

37. Bookman A, Harrington M. Family caregivers: a shadow workforce in the geriatric health care system. J Health Polit Policy Law 2007;32(6):1005–41.

38. U.S. Department of Health & Human Services, Office of Inspector General (US DHHS OIG). States' requirements for Medicaid-funded personal care service attendants. OEI-07-05-00250. Washington, DC: US DHHS; 2006.
39. Phi & Direct Care Worker Association of North Carolina (PHI/DCWA-NC). Results of the 2007 national survey of state initiatives on the long-term care direct care workforce; 2007.
40. Stone RI, Dawson S. The origins of better jobs better care. Gerontologist 2008; 48(Special Issue 1):5–13.
41. Bryant N, Stone RI. The role of state policy in developing the long-term care workforce. Generations, in press.
42. McDonald I, Davis G. The SEIU 775 long-term care training, support, and career development network: a blue print for the future. New York: PHI & 1199 SEIU Training & Education Fund; 2007.
43. Reinhard SC. Consumer-directed care and nurse practice acts. Washington, DC: Assistant Secretary for Planning and Evaluation, USDHHS, paper prepared for the National Symposium on Consumer Direction and Self-Determination for the Elderly and People with Disabilities; 2001.

Elder Abuse and Neglect: When Home Is Not Safe

L. Abbey, MD*

KEYWORDS

• Elder abuse • Elder neglect • Home visits • Geriatric

CASE SUMMARIES

1. Mrs. D. is an 80-year-old hemiplegic, aphasic homebound woman. She is cared for by her daughter and has always been up in a chair, neatly dressed and groomed for home visits. She generally smiles, nods, and shakes her head in response to questions. Today, she is still in bed in a rumpled but dry nightgown. Her daughter comes in briefly to say how hard it is now for her, since she has 2 small grandchildren to care for fulltime. She then goes into the next room and yells at the children to stop running around. The patient is frowning, and she will not raise her eyes to look up. Her examination is otherwise unchanged from baseline.

2. Mr. E. is a 72-year-old man with a history of stroke whose blood pressure has been very high on recent visits. The dosage of his antihypertensive medication has been increased recently, but today the patient says that he has not had any medications in over 2 weeks. The nephew with whom he lives, he says, has not been able to pick them up. He says his nephew works hard and is in poor health. The nephew does not return phone calls or respond to messages or letters.

3. Mrs. F. is an 85-year-old bedbound woman whose caregiver husband is very compulsive. He requires a 2-week notice to schedule home visits, and then sets up the exact time for visits, refusing to open the door if care providers come at any other time. The patient has always appeared well cared for, though she talks very little. Today the husband calls to report that the patient cries out whenever he attempts to turn her in bed and even when he just touches her left leg. Although he at first refuses, he eventually agrees to a mobile x-ray visit, and a spiral fracture of the left femur is identified.

4. Mr. G. is a 68-year-old blind man with diabetes mellitus, heart failure, and bilateral lower-leg amputations; he lives with a daughter. The house is in poor repair and is cluttered. A child, aged 11 years, comes in and asks if she can help, saying the

---

Primary Care/Geriatrics, Virginia Commonwealth University, Richmond, VA, USA
* House Calls Program, Virginia Commonwealth University, 1300 E. Marshall Street, PO Box 980102, Richmond, VA 23298.
E-mail address: labbey@mcvh-vcu.edu

Clin Geriatr Med 25 (2009) 47–60
doi:10.1016/j.cger.2008.10.003
0749-0690/08/$ – see front matter © 2009 Elsevier Inc. All rights reserved.

care-giving daughter is taking a nap. The patient says his daughter is limited in her thinking but kind to him. He does not want to live anywhere else. On examination, he is found to be thin and disheveled, and has a stage-2 sacral pressure ulcer. He does well on mental status screening.

5. Mrs. H. is an 80-year-old woman with dementia who lives with her grandson. When her confusion worsened, her grandson moved in with her from another state to provide care but is rarely seen by home care visitors. The personal care aide in the home says she has often had to stay late because he did not return at the time she needed to leave. There have been multiple aides who declined to return because of the grandson's angry outbursts. He has no known telephone number at work and does not answer cell phone messages. On this visit, the patient appears unusually agitated and restless. She has bruising under her left eye and around both wrists. Her mouth appears dry, and she refuses to take anything by mouth, which is also unusual for her.

6. Mrs. I. is a 92-year-old woman who has been brought to the emergency room (ER) by a granddaughter for a persistent cough. She has not been seen in that ER previously and has no records there. The granddaughter reports that the patient has a history of dysphagia but has declined a workup and has been losing weight over the past few months. The patient is thin and frail but alert, stating emphatically that she is fine and just wants "to go home." She is noted to have scattered bruises and skin tears over the backs of her hands and forearms. She refuses much of the physical examination, gives her name and address correctly, and then refuses to answer any further questions.

7. Mr. J. is a 75-year-old bed-bound man admitted to the hospital with bacteremia associated with a stage-4 pressure ulcer. His caregiver wife says she promised him he would never go to a nursing home, but she is clearly exhausted by the demands of caring for him. When asked how often she turns him, she says, "Whenever I can." There are no living children, and family supports are few. She thinks he makes too much money for government assistance but says they cannot afford to pay for custodial help. The patient is improving and is ready for discharge on home intravenous (IV) therapy.

INTRODUCTION

Since the first reports of elder abuse appeared in the medical literature more than 30 years ago,[1] studies from various disciplines—medical, nursing, social work, and law enforcement—have attempted to define the problem. While complex related issues are being debated and interventions evaluated, the importance of the problem and need for identifying elders at risk are clear.

The uniqueness of the patient's home as the site of care has important implications for detecting and managing elder abuse and neglect. Both family and paid caregivers are more likely to be present during a home visit than an office or hospital encounter, and the interaction between patient and caregiver can be observed. Suspicions can be corroborated or diminished during visits, discussion can be undertaken with others entering the home (aides, therapists), and observations can be made over time. The need for support services, caregiver respite, or even emergency protection from harm can be overt, or signs can be subtle and require a long-term relationship to identify. Because of frequent involvement with multiple disciplines during the provision of medical care, home care providers are often familiar with the myriad services that can be necessary for an adequate response.

PREVALENCE AND IMPORTANCE

Research on elders living in Europe, Canada, and the United States consistently indicates a 2% to 10% rate of elder abuse.[2-4] Despite mandatory reporting laws and greater public awareness in the medical literature and lay press, elder abuse is still underreported. According to the National Center on Elder Abuse, only 1 of 14 domestic adult abuse cases is reported.[5] Multiple studies have identified elder abuse as a worldwide problem.[6-12] An estimated 1.5 to 2 million older adults are neglected or abused in the United States annually.[13,14]

Abused elders are more likely to report serious health problems,[15] and elder abuse is a risk factor for nursing home placement.[16] Most importantly, those experiencing elder abuse and neglect have a high mortality rate.[17]

DEFINITION OF ELDER ABUSE AND NEGLECT

Although various definitions have been developed, separating physical, psychological, or financial acts (commissions) from omissions, a general definition is "intentional actions that cause harm or a serious risk of harm to a vulnerable elder by a caregiver or person who stands in a trust relationship with the elder, or failure by a caregiver to satisfy the elder's basic needs or to protect the elder from harm."[2] It is important to consider the many forms these acts or omissions can take and to be aware of subtle signs of abuse and neglect. Self-neglect is especially complex.

IDENTIFICATION

Private interviews of patient and caregiver should be arranged if possible. This may require some maneuvering if the home is modest. It is appropriate to ask the patient if he or she would like a private interview on all visits, so that this becomes the routine rather than an uncomfortable exception. Caregiver response may be observed; unusual reluctance may increase suspicion. A continuing relationship with the elder is important for obtaining information about a sensitive subject. Intense denial and embarrassment are typical in victims of abuse by relatives. Consider the cultural context and attempt to avoid alienating the patient and family. The caregiver's educational and skill level should be considered. The expected level of care would be different if the caregiver is a well-intentioned neighbor or even a frail elderly spouse, compared with a certified personal care aide or nurse. The challenge is to detect abuse and neglect without undermining a dedicated caregiver's continued help.

Abused patients may have a pattern of frequent provider changes or infrequent health maintenance visits, canceled visits, and vague or inconsistent details of injuries. "It is very common for victims to move back and forth between acknowledging and denying mistreatment or accepting and refusing assistance."[18]

Chronic diseases can mask or mimic elder abuse. Abuse should be considered if there is a peculiar pattern of injuries (hands, scalp, or face), wrist and ankle scars that suggest restraint use, poor hygiene, malnutrition, misuse or absence of medications, or poorly controlled chronic medical problems despite an apparently adequate medical plan. Multiple bruises of different colors typify child abuse but are less specific in the elderly.[19] Unusual locations of bruises or burns are of more concern. Long-bone fractures may indicate abuse but also may occur with minimal trauma.[20,21] Pressure ulcers, if not a result of unavoidable decline, and extensive skin tears can also indicate mistreatment. Documentation of findings should be detailed, including diagrams and photographs if feasible, since advocacy may involve court proceedings.

Signs of psychological abuse, which can include verbal harassment, belittling, threatening, and scolding, may be subtle. They can include withdrawal, apathy, rapid worsening of cognitive function, or new repetitive movements. Since many of these signs have a long differential diagnosis in geriatrics, a comprehensive approach is necessary, and full assessment may require several home visits.

Financial abuse is under-recognized and involves breaking trust by a manipulative or exploitive action, causing the elder to lose assets. This can involve contractors, salespersons, attorneys, paid caregivers, insurance agents, clergy, family, or friends.

Sexual abuse should be considered if genital or breast injuries are present. Elders are often reluctant to admit this has occurred. In some jurisdictions, suspicion of sexual abuse may require reporting to both law enforcement and social service officials.

Neglect can be intentional failure to provide goods and services necessary for optimal health and safety or unintentional and related to lack of resources and knowledge. Psychological neglect includes failure to provide social stimulation, isolation, and restricted socialization. Financial neglect can be failure to use available funds for needed goods and services for an elder's health and safety (including preserving the inheritance rather than spending it on elder care).

The distinction between, on the one hand, unfortunate but unavoidable events in the lives of frail elders or normal interpersonal stress and, on the other hand, abuse, is not always clear. While making a home visit, the provider can observe patient-caregiver interaction to obtain more insight. One strategy is to ask the caregiver to transfer the patient from bed to chair for the examination and observe the process.

Signs of an overburdened caregiver include impatience or anger directed toward the elder, excessive concern about treatment costs, focusing on the caregiver's own problems rather than the elder's, and asking for extra help. Interestingly, studies do not show that degree of caregiver stress correlates with abuse potential.[22] Abuse may relate to added stressors, such as poor financial situation, substance abuse, or long-term poor family relationships.

It is essential to consider cultural differences in judgments about possible elder abuse or neglect. Moon and Williams[23] found that people from different ethnic backgrounds interpreted the same scenarios of possible abuse or neglect differently, though extremes of abuse are apparent regardless of ethnicity. For more subtle situations, obtain information about cultural context, using nonfamily translators if needed.

The obligation of the home care provider is to have a high index of suspicion for what is an unfortunately common and under-recognized problem, screen for it, and refer when appropriate. Continue an established relationship, if possible, for medical support and assistance during the investigation.

RISK FACTORS FOR ELDER ABUSE

Although identifying possible risk factors helps focus attention, note that anyone— family member, paid caregiver, or unrelated person—can be an abuser and any elder—competent or incompetent, healthy or frail, male or female—can be a victim of abuse.

Elderly patients living alone are in most danger not just from direct caregivers but also from unscrupulous neighbors, salespersons, repairmen, and telephone or Internet scams.[24] A community survey in New Haven, CT,[2] identified risk factors as non-white race, age older than 75 years, difficulty/inability to eat, and poor social network. Another study[25] identified risk factors as low income, minority status, advanced age, substance abuse by elder or caregiver, prior history of abuse, and cognitive impairment. The extent of physical impairment is not necessarily associated with risk for abuse. Women are more commonly abused and are the victims in nearly all reported sexual abuse in elders.[26] The abuser is often male and the primary caregiver.[27] In one study,[22] abusive caregivers were more likely than other caregivers to have stopped working to care for the elder. Abuse is more likely within relationships that are already poor, and the elder may also be the abuser. Although a combative elder may precipitate an abusive exchange, reporting requirements may still mandate reporting. Possible contributing factors to abuse include parents taking deinstitutionalized mentally ill adult children back into the home, financial problems, patterns of intergenerational violence, and dependence of the caregiver on the elder for housing or financial resources.

REPORTING

All 50 states have elder abuse prevention laws with mandatory reporting when an elder is in an institution; most also require reporting when abuse occurs in a private home. Health care professionals are positioned to identify elder abuse and are mandated reporters in most states. Clinicians should know their state's reporting requirements. Not all states require reporting self-neglect. Reports are confidential, and the reporter is protected from litigation unless malicious intent is proven. Some states have penalties for failure to report. Most have a toll-free hotline telephone number. Information about state laws, resources, and toll-free numbers is on the National Center for Elder Abuse Web site.[5]

Adult Protective Services (APS) agencies receive and investigate reports of suspected elder abuse. The APS program was established under Title XX of the Social Security Act in 1975, federally mandated with little funding.[28] APS programs developed separately and so vary from state to state. Most cover both older and younger vulnerable adults. Vulnerable means the adult is unable to protect himself or herself because of age or disability. APS actions include receiving reports, assessing risk, evaluating decision-making capacity, and case planning. APS may also arrange for medical, social, financial, legal, housing, law enforcement, or other emergency or support services.

A 2004 survey of state APS programs funded by the Administration on Aging[29] showed a 19.7% increase in reports of elder and vulnerable adult abuse and neglect compared with a 2000 survey. Substantiated cases increased 15.6%. More than 40% of victims were aged 80 years or older. Alleged perpetrators included adult children (32.6%), other family members (21.5%), or spouse/intimate partners (11.3%). Clients refused services 16.0% of the time.

Most common reporters for older adults were family members (17.0%), social services (10.6%), friends/neighbors (8.0%), self (6.3%), long-term care staff (5.5%), law enforcement (5.3%), and nurses/aides (3.8%). Physicians constituted 1.4% of reporters.

Low Physician Reporting

Physicians infrequently report to APS agencies, although many see elderly patients on a regular basis. Possible reasons may include the following:

1. The physician may defer to others (social worker, nurse) to report
2. Lack of awareness of the problem
3. Lack of training in screening and interventions
4. Concern about losing relationship with the family

5. Denial that this family can be abusing—especially if other family members are also patients of the physician
6. Reluctance to be involved in legal and court proceedings
7. Time pressures prevent case finding
8. Concern about safety and fear of involvement
9. Signs of elder abuse may mimic other common illnesses in the elderly

Reluctance to consider abuse may come from concerns about potential negative outcomes if suspicions are incorrect or even more negative outcomes if they are correct. In one study of primary care physicians and perceived challenges in relation to mandatory reporting laws,[30] conflicting goals and paradoxes of improved or impaired physician-patient rapport, issues of patient quality of life, and physician control or ability to decide what is in the best interest of the patient were identified.

Physicians may be uncomfortable with the topic. "Family violence does not fit neatly within the traditional medical paradigm of symptoms, diagnoses and treatment."[31]

The social context may also be so complex that the best interest of the elder can be difficult to ascertain, especially if there is cognitive impairment or the elder refuses assistance: "However pathologic the relationship, severing the tie is always serious."[32] In spite of the challenges, clinicians should know and follow reporting laws.

LOW VICTIM SELF-REPORTING

Self-reporting by victims is also relatively low. Some possible reasons for this, which should be considered by clinicians working with the elderly, include the following:

1. Isolation, with no access to report
2. No knowledge of available resources
3. Denial of the problem
4. Embarrassment/shame at being in an abusive situation
5. Fear of retaliation by the abuser
6. Fear of nursing home placement
7. Poor self-esteem and feeling that abuse is deserved
8. Cognitive impairment

These reasons should be remembered when an elder is interviewed. A patient and empathic attitude, plus direct questioning, especially in the context of an ongoing relationship, may encourage a positive response. Nonverbal cues can also arouse suspicions if the elder does not acknowledge abuse directly or if a private interview is difficult to arrange.

SCREENING FOR ELDER ABUSE AND NEGLECT

There have been several proposed screening tools for elder abuse and neglect,[33–37] though none are in as common use as those screening for mental status,[38] activities of daily living,[39] or geriatric depression.[40] It may be best to begin with a general question: "How are things going for you here at home?" Any negative comments or suggestive nonverbal behaviors can be followed by more specific questions, which may include the following:

1. Has anyone at home ever hurt or threatened you?
2. Has anyone made you feel guilty about asking for help?
3. Has anyone refused to give you food or needed medicine?
4. Have you ever been asked to sign papers you did not understand?

5. Has anyone taken something from you without asking?
6. Has anyone touched you without your permission?

Interview the caregiver separately from the elder, if possible, because the caregiver may feel more able to talk about difficult care issues when the elder is not listening. General questions about how the situation is going can then move on to more specific areas of need. Support services may allow a burdened but dedicated caregiver to continue providing care and help avoid unintentional neglect from caregiver failure.

INTERVENTIONS FOR ELDER ABUSE AND DOMESTIC VIOLENCE IN LATE LIFE

Traditional emphasis of APS agencies has been on services and support for care-givers. Although increasing disability and care needs do not necessarily increase abuse, research shows that overburdened caregivers are more likely to abuse a dependent elder, especially if the relationship has been poor.[41] In these cases, care-giver education, support groups, respite, additional paid help in the home, and use of daycare can relieve pressure and stabilize a deteriorating situation.

Older women experience domestic violence well into old age. A common reason for abuse in later life may be power and control dynamics, similar to battering of younger victims.[42] Abusers may be spouses or partners, adult children, or other family members or caregivers. "In these cases the abuser feels a sense of entitlement to use various forms of abuse to gain and maintain power and control over the victim."[42]

Appropriate interventions differ with the situation. Adding services will not address control issues. In that case, safety planning, legal advocacy, information about dynamics of domestic violence for victim and abuser, and holding abusers accountable are the key strategies. These interventions are less available to older victims, especially those who are homebound or cognitively impaired. Increasing efforts are made to add resources. For example, the first Elder Abuse Forensic Center was established in 2003 by the Program in Geriatrics at the University of California, Irvine.[43] Few shelters can accommodate frail elders, although that need is also beginning to be addressed. One example is the Weinberg Center of the Hebrew Home for the Aged at Riverdale in the Bronx, NY.[41] Additionally, some states have changed domestic violence orders of protection to include "caregiver" in the definition of a domestic relationship.

When cognitive impairment exists, the situation is even more complex. Powers of attorney, conservatorships, and guardianships are legal options if victims are incapable of decision making. Clinicians then provide information about decision-making ability.

Although an older victim of abuse who is cognitively intact may not wish reporting to occur, mandated reporting laws require it. In these situations, involvement of law enforcement to protect the elder may be necessary.

Involvement of law enforcement in elder abuse is developing. In the past, crimes committed in one's own home against another family member have been viewed somewhat differently from crimes by strangers.[44] Families have been allowed to work with social services agencies and preserve the family unit. "In serious cases, the criminal justice system may provide the only way to protect the vulnerable elder."[45]

SELF-NEGLECT

Self-neglect is the most common reason for APS referral in the National Center for Elder Abuse (NCEA) 2004 APS survey.[29] Because of its prevalence and the tension between respect for autonomy and self-determination and mandatory reporting laws, plus perceptual and cultural differences between health care providers and some elders, this situation warrants further discussion.

Self-neglect is a spectrum of behaviors characterized by inattention to health and hygiene and inability or unwillingness to access services.[46] Some self-neglect is relatively trivial, such as amassing piles of newspapers or more extensive hoarding.[47] Others can be dangerous, such as poor lighting, loss of utility service for nonpayment of bills, lack of medication refills, presence of spoiled food, presence of animal feces, and insect infestations.

In a study of self-neglecting elders who had been found living in squalor and admitted to the hospital, diagnoses included dementia, depression, and psychosis.[48] Other contributors include obsessive-compulsive disorder, alcoholism, or other substance abuse. Geriatric assessment of self-neglecting elderly found "executive dyscontrol" leading to functional impairment in a setting of inadequate medical and social support.[49] The seriousness of self-neglect is shown by a 13-year longitudinal study of elders with twice the risk of death within 3 years of APS investigation for self-neglect.[17]

Home care providers are positioned to identify isolated elders, provide medical care, and arrange support. This can be challenging; denial is common and initial refusal to change is typical. Evaluation should be comprehensive, including detailed medical, psychiatric, functional, and social history, ideally by an interdisciplinary team. Evaluation of decision-making capacity is crucial but may be limited by funding and circumstances. Cognitive impairment can develop gradually, and ability to state preferences can persist even after an elder cannot manage complicated issues such as personal finances. Self-neglecting elders living alone may have no close family or friends or may be alienated.

Remember that elders sometimes make choices that health care providers, family members, and friends disagree with. This may relate to limited options such as nursing home placement, a drastic change after living for decades in the same familiar home and neighborhood. Sometimes after recognition, reporting, investigation, and intervening to the extent possible or acceptable, the elder remains in a suboptimal situation. Home care providers can remain involved, encouraging appropriate decisions, working with the support network, educating about health and safety needs, coordinating medical care, community services, and protection from financial and other abuses, and being available when intervention is ultimately mandatory. This may occur urgently. When social interventions are required, seek the least disruptive alternative. At these transitions, continued involvement of the home care team offers support and continuity. "Americans are fiercely independent, a highly valued personal trait respected by most health care professionals. In some instances, however, when older persons no longer can care for themselves, then personal health, well-being, and even their lives are at risk."[50]

PROVIDER ROLE IN ELDER ABUSE AND NEGLECT

Individual judgment dictates how much evidence is needed to warrant reporting suspected elder abuse or neglect. Clinicians should know their state's laws and community supports. Preventive strategies include screening for substance abuse and dementia, educating and counseling caregivers, and referring to support groups, local Alzheimer's Association chapters, Area Agencies on Aging, financial counselors, legal aid, and elder law specialists. Involving home care resources and addressing stressful problems like incontinence and disruptive behavior help as do respite and adult daycare.

Be aware of family violence. Identify local resources and safe shelters. Involve law enforcement when there is immediate danger to the elder or if the clinician feels threatened. Depending on time and interests, health care professionals may be actively involved in advocacy for funding of services. As states expand mandated reporter lists, funding for education and referral procedures should be pursued.

As much as home care providers can assist in identifying elder abuse and neglect, they can enter homes only with permission. There are elders who are victims and live in isolation. Clinicians can be involved in education of communities and those who may have contact with homebound elders: delivery and cable personnel, maintenance staff in apartment buildings, employees of financial institutions, and others. An algorithm for elder abuse screening and intervention is available.[35]

SUMMARY

The complex phenomenon of elder abuse and neglect requires collaboration of home care professionals with other disciplines, including social services, law enforcement, and legal support. Identification can be challenging, but the prevalence suggests that routine screening may be advisable. Knowing and working effectively with local resources is important. "Protecting older people, assisting in creative interventions and developing needed services is a shared professional responsibility."[45]

CASE DISCUSSIONS
Case 1

Changes in caregiver demands can cause a dedicated caregiver to become overwhelmed, and care of the elder can deteriorate into neglect or abuse. Warning signs here include new responsibilities of the caregiver, her lack of attention to the patient and the provider, and her comments being more about herself than the patient. Subtle signs from the patient are change in behavior (not up and dressed as usual) and reluctance to look at the provider. This can indicate embarrassment about the caregiver or anger about the situation. Note that there are no other physical findings, so one must be alert. Yet, clearly, the situation is stressed and intervention needed. Depending on the home visitor's expertise and resources available, this could include a conversation with the daughter to assess her needs and provide support (additional care in the home or elsewhere for patient, children, or both; social worker to discuss placement options; referral to a support group). Often, burdened caregivers are relieved to have problems identified to obtain needed help. Contacting APS might be indicated if the daughter refuses to acknowledge a deteriorating situation and future visits, scheduled sooner than routine, show no improvement in the care-giving situation.

Case 2

This patient is at risk of another stroke and needs medications. The problem has likely been going on for longer than 2 weeks. Attempts to contact the caregiver, find lower cost sources of medications, and address unmet needs of the caregiver are appropriate first steps. In this case, the caregiver has not been available and potential harm can occur. APS referral is indicated. Referral is confidential, and the decision to tell the patient about the referral would be up to the provider. It would be reasonable to question the elder further about other aspects of her health, safety, and finances, because multiple types of abuse and neglect may be present.

Case 3

Domestic violence can continue into older ages and can be difficult to identify when elders have impaired mobility and are isolated. Concerns related to this patient's husband include his apparent controlling nature and reluctance to have outsiders enter the home. The patient's lack of verbal expression may or may not be a concern. Up to this point, the care has seemed fine. It can be difficult to obtain a private conversation in the home, but this should be attempted. If the patient is cognitively intact, she should be offered assistance. The provider who best knows the caregiver may be best positioned to address issues. The fracture is troubling. Fractures can occur in long-time immobilized patients with minimal trauma,[20,21] but separate histories should be obtained from patient and caregiver if possible. If suspicious, mandated reporters may be obligated to make an APS report for social work to gain access to the home. Although reports are anonymous, the husband may infer that the referral came from the physician thus effectively severing the relationship with the couple. If the caregiver resists obtaining proper treatment including pain management, it may be best to recommend an ER visit. If the caregiver seems appropriately concerned and willing to follow needed care plans, it may be preferable to maintain the relationship and make no APS referral to preserve a role in continuing care.

Case 4

Self-neglect is a common cause for APS referral. Because elders vary in what they accept, defining self-neglect can be difficult. In addition, an elder who is cognitively intact can refuse help at home or placement. This does not remove the obligation to report. The referral can be explained as a legal obligation and also an opportunity to obtain assistance. Social needs could improve with a volunteer financial or legal aide. Many communities have volunteers who repair homes. Home health referral for wound care could provide a home safety assessment and social work support. APS cannot remove someone from their situation (no protective custody, unlike child protective services) or initiate services if the cognitively intact elder refuses, but APS can provide support services and in-home psychiatric assessment of decision-making capacity. Since the home visit is during school hours, presence of a school-aged child may warrant calling Child Protective Services.

Case 5

Involvement of law enforcement in addition to APS is appropriate when the patient is in imminent danger. This is a judgment call but is important to pursue if appropriate because of the increased mortality in elders referred to APS.[17] Concerns in this case include a largely unknown caregiver who depends on the patient at least for housing, reports of verbal abuse, failure to return calls, and evidence of injury on the patient. Given findings of decreased intake and possible dehydration, ambulance transport to an ER is appropriate. Summoning the police during this process would protect the provider if the caregiver returns unexpectedly and resists the process. APS could be contacted to be included in hospital discharge planning. The home care provider should stay in contact with the hospital staff about the home situation so that the problem is addressed. With cognitive impairment, legal support may be needed for guardianship proceedings.

Case 6

Continuity of care is indispensable in medical care for frail elders. Without background information, accurate assessment of medical and social situations is difficult. If possible, the patient's primary care or other previous provider should be contacted to obtain appropriate information. This would include decision-making capacity, prior discussions about medical workup and treatment goals, and family support. The ER provider should still evaluate her current mental status and ability to make the decision to refuse treatment. The skin tears and bruises may simply result from having aged fragile skin[19] but should be documented. Evidence of other apparent injuries and the interaction between patient and family member should be observed. A social work consultation in the ER may help to explore support needs, because the ER visit could primarily reflect caregiver stress rather than an ill patient. If the patient is judged as able to refuse services but seems to need further medical care, APS may need to be contacted. In any case, she needs close follow-up, and a home visit could be very helpful.

Case 7

Many frail elders are cared for by equally frail spouses who can become overwhelmed by caregiving with negative outcomes for both. If the patient has had home health visits for wound care, the nurses can be an excellent source of information about the care environment. Adding home IV therapy to an already stressed situation is ill advised. There may be other family or friends who can be recruited to help, and family finances should be re-evaluated. Short-term nursing facility admission may be acceptable even if long-term placement is not. APS may supply urgent in-home assistance if the final decision is to return home. A home health agency social worker would then be helpful.

RESOURCES

National Center for Elder Abuse (NCEA)—established by US Administration on Aging, and disseminates information to professionals and the public; provides technical assistance and training to states and community organizations. Web site lists abuse hotlines, support services, state resources, research, statistics, publications, and legal aspects. 1225 Eye St. NW suite 725, Washington, DC 20005, 202-898-2586. Available at: www.elderabusecenter.org.

Clearinghouse on Abuse and Neglect of the Elderly (CANE)—located at the University of Delaware, archive of published research, training resources, government documents, and other resources on elder abuse. Department of Consumer Studies and Research, University of Delaware, 297 Graham Hall, Newark, DE 19716, 302-831-3525. Available at: www.cane.udel.edu.

Elder Locator—sponsored by the Administration on Aging; if given address and zip code of elder at risk, Elder Locator can refer caller to appropriate local agency to report abuse. 1-800-677-1116.

National Domestic Violence Hotline—available 24 hours a day, 365 days a year. 1-800-799-SAFE; TDD 1-800-787-3224.

REFERENCES

1. Burstone G. Granny bashing. [letter]. Br Med J 1975;3:592.
2. Lachs MS, Pillmer K. Elder abuse. Lancet 2004;364:1263–72.
3. Ogg T, Bennett G. Elder abuse in Britain. Br Med J 1992;305:998–9.
4. Podnieks E. The victimization of older persons. Can J Psychiatr Nurs 1987;28: 6–11.

5. Tatara T, Kuzmeskus LM. Trends in elder abuse in domestic settings. National Center on Elder Abuse Grant no. 90-am-0660. Washington, DC; May 1996. Available at: http://ncea.aoa.gov/ncearoot/Main_Site/Index.aspx. Accessed June 18, 2008.

6. Sharon N, Zoabi S. Elder abuse in a land of tradition; the case of Israeli's Arabs. J Elder Abuse Negl 1997;8:43–58.

7. Saveman B, Hallberg I, Norberg A, et al. Patterns of abuse of the elderly in their own homes as reported by district nurses. Scand J Prim Health Care 1993;11: 111–6.

8. Yan E, Tang C. Elder abuse by caregivers: a study of prevalence and risk factors in Hong Kong Chinese families. J Fam Violence 2004;19:269–77.

9. Malley-Morrison K, Nyryan E. International perspective on elder abuse: five case studies. Educ Gerontol 2006;32:1–11.

10. Rinsky K, Malley-Morrison K. Russian perspectives on elder abuse: an exploratory study. J Elder Abuse Negl 2006;18:123–39.

11. Daskalopoulos MD, Kbouros A, Stathopoulou G. Perspectives on elder abuse in Greece. J Elder Abuse Negl 2006;18:87–104.

12. Mercurio AE, Nyborn J. Cultural definitions of elder maltreatment in Portugal. J Elder Abuse Negl 2006;18:51–65.

13. Aravanis SC. Diagnostic and treatment guidelines on elder abuse and neglect. Arch Fam Med 1993;2:371–88.

14. US Congress. House Select Committee on aging. Elder abuse: what can be done?. Washington, DC: United States Government Printing Office; 1991.

15. Fish BS, Regal SL. Extent and frequency of abuse in the lives of older women. Gerontologist 2002;42:200–9.

16. Lachs MS, Williams CS, O'Brien S, et al. Adult protective service use and nursing home placement. Gerontologist 2002;42:734–9.

17. Lachs MS, Williams CS, O'Brien S, et al. The mortality of elder mistreatment. JAMA 1998;280:428–32.

18. Bloom JS, Ansell P, Bloom MN. Detecting elder abuse: a guide for physicians. Geriatrics 1989;44:40–4, 56.

19. Mosqueda L, Burnight K, Liao S. The life cycle of bruises in older adults. J Am Geriatr Soc 2005;53:1339–43.

20. Kane RS, Goodwin JS. Spontaneous fracture of the long bones in nursing home patients. Am J Med 1991;90:263–6.

21. Miyusaka Y, Sakurai M, Yokobori AT Jr, et al. Bending and torsion fractures in long bones (a mechanical and radiologic assessment of clinical cases). Biomed Mater Eng 1991;1:3–10.

22. Homer AC, Gilleard C. Abuse of elderly people by the carers. Br Med J 1990;301: 1359–62.

23. Moon A, Williams O. Perceptions of elder abuse and help-seeking patterns among African-American, Caucasian-American, and Korean-American elderly women. Gerontologist 1993;33:386–95.

24. Lachs M, Pillmer K. Abuse and neglect of elderly persons. N Engl J Med 1995; 332:437–43.

25. Comijs HC, Smit JH, Pot AM, et al. Risk indicators of elder mistreatment in the community. J Elder Abuse Negl 1998;9:67–76.

26. Epplin J. Clinical Q&A: identifying elder abuse in the home care setting. Ann Long Term Care 2006;14:15–6.

27. Ramsey-Klawsnik H. Elder abuse offenders: a typology. Generations 2000;2: 17–22.

28. About Adult Protective Services. National Center on elder Abuse website. Available at: http://ncea.aoa.gov/NCEAroot/Main_Site/Find_Help/APS/About_APS.aspx. Accessed June 18, 2008.
29. The 2004 survey of state adult protective services: abuse of adults 60 years of age and older. Washington, DC: National Center on Elder Abuse; 2006. Available at: http://www.aspnetwork.org/resources/docs/AbuseAdults60.pdf. Accessed June 19, 2008.
30. Rodriguez MA, Wallace SP, Woolf NH, et al. Mandatory reporting of elder abuse: between a rock and a hard place. Ann Fam Med 2006;4:403–9.
31. Walling A. Interventions and treatment strategies for elder abuse. Am Fam Physician 2005;72:896–7.
32. Rosenblatt DE. Elder abuse: what can physicians do? Arch Fam Med 1996;5:88–90.
33. Ansell P, Breckman R. Elder mistreatment guidelines for health care professionals: detection, assessment, and intervention. New York: Mount Sinai/Victim Services Agency; 1988.
34. Aravanis SC, Adelman RD, Breckman R, et al. Diagnostic and treatment guidelines on elder abuse and neglect. Chicago (IL): American Medical Association; 1992.
35. Nelson HD, Nygren P, McInerney Y, et al. Screening women and elderly adults for family and intimate partner violence: a review of the evidence for the US Preventive Services Task Force. Ann Intern Med 2004;140:387–96.
36. Fulmer T, Wetle T. Elder abuse screening and intervention. Nurse Pract 1986;11:33–8.
37. Hwalek MA, Sengstock MC. Assessing the probability of abuse of the elderly toward development of a clinical screening instrument. J Appl Gerontol 1986;5:153–73.
38. Folstein MF, Folstein SE, McHugh PR. Mini mental state: a practical method for grading the cognitive state of patients for the clinician. J Psychiatr Res 1975;12:189–98.
39. Katz S, Ford AB, Moskowitz RW, et al. Studies of illness in the aged: the index of ADL: a standardized measure of biological and psychological function. JAMA 1963;185:914–9.
40. Yesavage JA, Brink TL, Rose TL, et al. Development and validation of a geriatric depression rating scale: a preliminary report. J Psychiatr Res 1983;17:37–49.
41. Reingold DA. An elder abuse shelter program: build it and they will come, a long term care based program to address elder abuse in the community. J Gerontol Soc Work 2006;46:123–35.
42. Brandl B. Assessing for abuse in later life. National clearinghouse on abuse in later life. Available at: http://www.ncall.us. 2004; Accessed July 3, 2008.
43. Wiglesworth A, Mosqueda L, Burnight K, et al. Findings from an elder abuse forensic center. Gerontologist 2006;46:277–83.
44. Bergeron LR. Self-determination and elder abuse: do we know enough? J Gerontol Soc Work 2006;46:81–102.
45. Heisler C. The role of the criminal justice system in elder abuse cases. J Elder Abuse Negl 1991;3:5–33.
46. Pavlou MP, Lachs MS. Could self-neglect in older adults be a geriatric syndrome? J Am Geriatr Soc 2006;54:831–42.
47. Clark AN, Mandikar GD, Gray I. Diogenes' syndrome: a clinical study of gross neglect in old age. Lancet 1975;1:366–8.
48. MacMillan D, Shaw P. Senile breakdown in standards of personal and environmental cleanliness. Br Med J 1966;2:1032–7.

49. Dyer CB, Goodwin JS, Pickens-Pace S, et al. Self-neglect among the elderly: a model based on more than 500 patients seen by a geriatric medicine team. Am J Public Health 2007;97:1671–6.
50. Dyer CB, Pickens S, Burnett J. Vulnerable elders: when it is no longer safe to live alone. JAMA 2007;298:1440–50.

Assistive Technologies in the Home

Kenneth Brummel-Smith, MD*, Mariana Dangiolo, MD

KEYWORDS

- Assistive technology • Home care • Rehabilitation • Walkers
- Safety devices • Wheelchairs • Smart homes

EPIDEMIOLOGY OF DISABILITY

Although the rapid growth of the older population is familiar, the fact that the aged will soon be baby boomers presents special challenges. Though the rate of incident disability is decreasing, the numeric increase in old people will mean that many more persons with disability will be receiving home care services.[1] The Administration on Aging projects that 19% of adults 65 years and older will have some limitation in performing activities of daily living (ADLs), and 4% will have severe disability associated with aging.[2] In fact 95% of our elders currently live in private residences.[3] More than 75% of older adults with disabilities use some type of assistive device.[4]

One promising solution to the needs of homebound elders with disability is the use of assistive technology (AT) devices to compensate for physical limitations. Their use has experienced growth far exceeding the demographic changes mentioned here. Currently, approximately one in four older adults uses an assistive device and one-third of those use more than one device.[5] Assistive devices reduce the task difficulty and the need for help from another person. Technology that can help seniors achieve their dream of living at home longer will provide a win-win effect, both improving quality of life and reducing health care expenditures.

AT is defined as "any item, piece of equipment, or product system, whether acquired commercially, modified, or customized, that is used to increase, maintain, or improve functional capabilities of individuals with disabilities."[6] This definition of AT is estimated to comprise more than 18,000 devices, items of durable medical equipment, and environmental modifications that are supplied by an industry of more than 2,000 companies.[7] Under this broad definition, AT ranges from low-tech items, such as canes, crutches, grab bars, and walkers, to high-tech equipment, such as speech synthesizers and power wheelchairs.[8]

The latter half of the twentieth century saw dramatic growth in AT use by older persons with disabilities. During the 1980s, the number using any equipment rose

Department of Geriatrics, 1115 West Call Street, Florida State University College of Medicine, Tallahassee, FL 32306-4300, USA
* Corresponding author.
E-mail address: ken.brummel-smith@med.fsu.edu (K. Brummel-Smith).

Clin Geriatr Med 25 (2009) 61–77
doi:10.1016/j.cger.2008.11.003
0749-0690/08/$ – see front matter © 2009 Elsevier Inc. All rights reserved.

from 3.3 to 4.1 million, and the number relying only on equipment more than doubled.[9] By the mid-1990s, most of those with ADL limitations used some form of technology, and almost a third (31%) used only AT to accommodate their needs.[10]

The subject of aging in America is becoming the focus of a new wave in health care engineering research: development of innovative assistive devices and "smart home" (SH) technologies that can be customized to individuals' needs and enhance self-worth, independence, safety, and mobility. Several concurrent population trends, such as increasing education levels in the older population, decreasing availability of informal caregivers, and a shrinking long-term care workforce, have led to discussions of the potential of AT to promote independent aging.[11]

It is hoped that use of AT can improve quality of life and alleviate pressures on the long-term care system. Recent national studies suggest that technology may confer unique benefits in reducing difficulty with daily tasks and unmet needs.[12–15] Yet it remains unclear whether AT replaces or supplements personal care. Where the use of AT reduces the amount of personal care needed, public expenditures on home health care could be reduced and burdens of informal care alleviated.[16] Alternatively, use of AT in addition to personal services could improve quality of care and perhaps prevent functional decline and institutionalization, which would also reduce public and private health care expenditures. The capacity of equipment to substitute for or to supplement personal care is task-specific and depends on the type of device and the personal care providers. In general, those using simple devices are less likely to use informal care, and those using complex devices are more likely to use formal care.[10]

Kraskowsky and colleagues[17] reviewed the literature on the factors affecting older adults' use of adaptive equipment. Between 47% and 82% of prescribed equipment continues to be used by older adults, with use decreasing over time. Findings from published studies show that equipment suitability, adequate training, and pre-prescription home visits contribute to these rates of use.

There are social, environmental, and emotional factors related to elders' use of devices. One cannot assume that an elder will use a product simply because he or she needs it. Many older persons choose to avoid social interactions rather than to be seen using a device that is aesthetically undesirable or embarrassing. Hence, it is essential to understand both the principles of assessing need and proper training in the use of AT.

PRINCIPLES OF THE USE OF AT

An assistive device is prescribed when a person has a diminished capacity to perform a function within a prescribed range. There are two other interventions for people with disabilities, which are not addressed in this article: adapting the techniques the person uses to accomplish the function and adapting the environment at large. While the former is an important part of rehabilitation, the latter is something that must often occur in tandem with the provision of many assistive technologies. For instance, doors may need to be widened for walkers, and ramps installed to allow wheelchairs to be used. For an extensive discussion on home modifications, see the Web site of the Center for Inclusive Design and Environmental Access[18] and the Center for Universal Design.[19]

Although any patient can buy a cane at a yard sale, the proper process for acquiring an assistive device is much more complex. It involves four important steps: (1) patient assessment, which shows that a disability exists that can be served by a device; (2) assessment of the patient's motivation to use a device; (3) collaborative, informed decision making between the patient and the health care professional about the type of device needed; and (4) training in the proper use of the device. As the patient is the one who will either use the device or store it in the closet, it is essential that the patient's goals and views are known. From the health care provider's view, devices can serve multiple purposes, such as energy conservation, allowing the patient to accomplish tasks he or she would not otherwise be able to do, preventing deterioration of function, or reducing risk of injury. In general, devices should increase patient independence. However, if the patient receives secondary gain from being assisted by a family member, no device is likely to be successfully used if it reduces the help from the caregiver.

A common issue encountered by geriatric practitioners is the concern that a device will increase dependence or reduce function. For instance, when in a progressive course of worsening mobility, should a person obtain a wheelchair? If provided too early, the normal conditioning mechanisms that occur while walking will be lost; too late, and the person may risk an adverse event, such as a fall, or social isolation. In general, it is best to err on the side of the patient's desire, as there is little evidence that wheelchairs are overused.[20] As Huxley said, "The will of the patient, not the health of the patient, is the ultimate goal of health care." Such a situation should be approached using informed consent. All devices, like medications, have potential side effects. The patient should receive the benefit of the professional's recommended action and the alternatives, with the risks and benefits of each, and what is likely to occur if no device is used.

Finally, during the assessment, it is important to establish a plan to review the use of the device, its proper maintenance, and changes in need over time. Even simple devices such as canes require maintenance. The failure of a rubber tip on the cane can lead to a disastrous fall. Complex devices such as powered wheelchairs or computerized medication dispensers may require weekly surveillance. If the patient's disabling condition is progressive, the device may need to be changed as new functional problems develop. All this complexity highlights the need for ongoing collaboration between the patient, the caregivers, and the homecare team.

Generally, these types of modifications and devices are obtained through a home health agency. While a home nurse, occupational therapist (OT), physical therapist (PT), or other type of provider may recommend an assistive device, a physician's order is usually required for it to be covered by Medicare. Accurate documentation is required. Often, patients who have a stay in a rehabilitation facility (hospital-based or in a skilled nursing facility) will be provided equipment. It is still best for the home care team to reassess the patient's need and training at home as the patient's functional abilities may have changed.

FEEDING AIDS

Adequate nutritional intake is critical to preserve the health of older people. Almost 50% of elderly people have inadequate intake of 1 or more nutrients, and 24% of those aged 85 years and older cannot feed independently. The ability to self-feed is typically the first ADL ability mastered as a child and the last to be lost as we become frail and deconditioned. Eating is also the most social of all ADLs, as dining is usually a shared experience. Therefore, full assessment of nutritional issues is multidimensional, interdisciplinary, and goes beyond our goals for this article. A nutritionist is very useful in assessing and recommending nutritional interventions. However, there are a number of assistive devices designed to facilitate independent feeding that should be discussed.[21]

In general, no universal guidelines link individual feeding devices to specific conditions; any one device can be helpful for multiple types of disability. Feeding aids should always be kept clean and readily available. If possible, they should look normal and attractive; otherwise, patients will not accept them. Occupational therapists can assess patients with specific feeding problems and provide a variety of devices to try. Currently, there is no objective evidence of their value, and recommending their use is based on empirical observation.

For patients with poor grip due to weakness, pain, or stiffness, lightweight utensils with large handles are good. Swivel utensils are effective for people with tremors, limited grasps, poor coordination, and/or upper-extremity weakness. Cutlery with detachable handles that clip to a plastic hand strap can be useful for people with weak finger flexion. Cognitive impairment can affect pronation as silverware is brought to the mouth. This problem may be solved using utensils that have a swivel handle, allowing the spoon or fork to remain level.[22]

Plates with sides, plastic plate guards, and rubberized place mats to prevent plates from sliding are useful to keep food on the plate and facilitate getting food onto the utensil. Cups with antisplash lids prevent spilling. Rocker knives eliminate the need to stabilize food with the other hand. Lightweight, insulated mugs prevent burns, and cups with two handles also help with poor grip. Prevention of dribbling can be achieved by using cups with spouts. For patients unable to suck fluids, straws with nonreturn valves often solve the problem. Patients with visual impairments will find large utensils with contrasting colors very useful.

ADAPTIVE CLOTHING AND DRESSING AIDS

Clothing, an integral part of self-identity and well-being, plays a key role in our daily social interactions. Dressing is affected by many chronic conditions that affect later life. Hobbs and Damon reported that 16% of persons 85 years and older have impairments in dressing.[23] Many elders with dressing difficulty find alternative ways to compensate for this disability, such as wearing slippers instead of shoes. This behavior may lead them to stay at home and experience further isolation. An occupational therapist can assess, recommend, and train the patient in the use of these devices or modifications.

Several problems can interfere with the dressing process, such as pain, decreased range of motion, or inability to make decisions on what to wear. Gender differences have also been reported. Mann and colleagues[24] observed that men when compared with women, more often, have lower-extremity dressing difficulties than upper-extremity difficulties.

Dressing aids and adaptive clothing can help people preserve their independence and retain control of their lives. Dressing sticks are wooden dowels, usually about 24 in long, with a coat hook inserted in the end. They can be used to pull off socks, unhook Velcro closures on shoes, or bring clothing over the shoulder. Buttonhooks are passed through the buttonhole, hooked over the button, and then the button is pulled into place. Stocking gutters and long-handled shoehorns may be used by people who have trouble donning socks or putting on shoes. Reachers are useful for people with fatigue and decreased mobility to pick up objects from the floor or other inaccessible locations.

For people with limited dexterity such as hand arthritis, clothing adaptations such as zippers with grab loops and touch fastener tape products, such as Velcro, that replace buttons, shoelaces, or zippers are useful. For incontinent patients, waistline side openings and long fly openings with zippers or touch fastener tape are recommended.

Side-zip pants or sweats with long zippers help patients with decreased hip or knee mobility and are excellent for non–weight-bearing patients. Back-flap pants are also good for patients who cannot stand or bear weight. One-piece jumpsuits and sweat sets also help patients who undress inappropriately. Arm and leg protectors prevent abrasion of the aged fragile skin. Foot deformities such as bunions and hammertoes require some adaptations that include deep toe box, plantar cushion, arch support, and lightweight shoes.

Dressing aids are widely available, simple to use, and relatively inexpensive, but as with other assistive devices, it is highly recommended that a thorough assessment of the patient first be conducted. Skilled professionals such as occupational therapists can individualize the patient's needs, provide appropriate training, and recommend special movements or positions that can make the dressing task much easier.

BATHING AND TOILETING DEVICES

Approximately 5% to 7% of community-living older adults require personal assistance with bathing, and more than one-third have difficulty bathing. Bathing disability is associated with many adverse consequences, such as a high incidence of falls and fractures, increased hospitalization, admission to skilled nursing facilities, and mortality. Many older persons simply give up on bathing or take sponge baths. However, dependency in bathing and toileting can be mitigated by using adaptive devices for the bathroom, improving quality of life and hygiene. If the patient has or is at risk of having bathing problems, he or she should be evaluated by both an occupational therapist and a PT.

Bathroom modifications to be considered include installation of grab bars to facilitate tub mobility and increase safety. A good hand grasp is required for the effective use of grab bars. Grab bars should be installed into studs on the walls to provide secure support and have a color that contrasts with the surface. Bar height and orientation are adjusted to patient need: for example, a vertical bar outside the tub can assist a person getting into the tub while standing, whereas lower bars help achieve balance when seated.

Access to a walk-in or wheel chair accessible shower stall is ideal for persons with bathing disability, but the cost of renovation may be prohibitive. Hence, many home dwelling elders will require modifications in the bathtub. Bath benches, rubber mats, and hydraulic lift bath seats address safe mobility. Bath stools or chairs are inexpensive and are reported to be among the most common devices used by elders at home.[25] These devices require good mobility to get in and out of the tub, and some of them lack back support, whereas other models have backrests and armrests or side rails that provide extra support. A transfer bench is ideal for people who need to transfer in a seated position, such as persons with a stroke. For persons with pronounced disability, lifts are available, but these are large, heavy, and costly.

The water thermostat should be set below 120° to prevent burns. Antiscald safety valves can be installed for this purpose. Flooring should be made slip-resistant using abrasive strips and nonskid mats. Safety treads provide a more permanent surface and are easier to clean. Bath mats are important for everyone who uses a bathtub, especially those who have lost strength and balance; mats have been associated with a 23% lower risk of persistent bathing disability.[26] Even though bath devices facilitate performing a key ADL task, we lack longitudinal studies to demonstrate the benefits of bath aids in promoting independent bathing in community-living older persons.

Raised toilet seats facilitate transfers for elders with impaired joints and balance problems. Alternatively, bars can be attached to the toilet seat bolts, or grab bars can be placed on the wall near the toilet. A combination of vertical and horizontal grab bars is ideal. There are models that swing down into place besides the toilet when needed but then can be lifted out of the way for people without disability.

Resistance to adoption has also been reported. As an example, grab bars are present only in 7% of older adult households.[27] Many studies that looked at attitudes and preferences about bathroom device use describe patient's feelings of embarrassment, denial of need, unsafe device use, lack of training on appropriate use, lack of access to services that install them, lack of funding for purchase, and vendor-related problems. For this reason, a systematic home assessment by a skilled professional can be helpful in providing an individualized selection of equipment, training, and adequate follow-up.

DEVICES FOR MOBILITY

Devices to promote mobility are probably the most commonly used AT. There are hundreds of different types of mobility devices. This discussion addresses technology for facilitating transfers, walking (canes and walkers), and wheeled mobility. In general, a PT is the health care provider most helpful in determining which type of device would best suit the patient and in the training for its use.

Canes are commonly acquired by patients without the benefit of an assessment by a PT. As a result they are often used incorrectly (on the wrong side, with improper advancement technique, or excessive weighting) and are usually too long. A properly fitted cane should extend to the crook of the wrist when the arm is hanging loosely at the patient's side. It should be used in the hand on the opposite side of the impaired leg and is advanced when the opposite leg is advanced. No more than 25% of the patient's body weight should be supported by the cane. Canes are best for people with stability problems from neuropathy (the additional upper-extremity neural input promotes better balance) or to reduce pain in an arthritic hip or knee. The end must have an intact rubber tip for safety. A single-point cane may be helpful in reducing falls in patients with Parkinson's disease (PD).[28] Some patients prefer a 4-prong cane because more weight can be applied. The main risk of this device is stability—all 4 prongs must be in solid contact with the ground once the patient's body weight is accepted.

Crutches are rarely used by older persons. Because of the excess stress placed on the wrists, a forearm attachment may be needed. Crutches are used mostly during initial rehabilitation after an amputation, but often the patient "graduates" to using a cane.

There are many types of walkers. The fit is the same as a cane, with the top of the handles at the crook of the wrist. The standard pickup walker (no wheels) is relatively useless because of complexity of use and the abnormal gait pattern produced. The common two-wheeled, front-wheel walker is helpful for patients who need to put more weight on the device than is safe with a cane. They are also helpful when patients have bilateral leg weakness or poor coordination and may also be helpful in PD patients with retropulsion. Front-wheeled walkers promote a more normal gait pattern than pickup walkers but can be difficult to maneuver in tight environments like mobile homes. The four-wheeled walker (with swiveling front wheels) promotes a much more normal gait pattern. It can be helpful in patients who have difficulty initiating gait (such as PD) but is risky in those with festination. These walkers are quite useful in patients with limited endurance, such as those with cardiac or pulmonary problems. Some models have brakes and a seat on which to rest. Good cognition and hand control are necessary to use these accessories safely. A Merry Walker is a four-wheeled walker/chair combination useful for someone who is at risk of falls. The person stands inside the walker and can sit down when desired on the internal seat. Doors in the house must be wide enough to accommodate its passage.

Wheelchairs are used when either the patient is unable to ambulate with a device or for longer distance travel in someone who would fatigue using a walker or cane. The type of wheelchair most health care providers are familiar with is not adequate for use as an independent mobility device. This is because most wheelchairs found in hospitals or doctors' offices are made for others to transport the patient. Personal wheelchairs must be fitted for the patient, and an almost infinite number of adaptations are possible.

For independent use a wheelchair must be lighter, have tip protection wheels on the back to prevent the user from performing a "wheelie," and a padded seat. Brakes must be easy to apply and footrests easy to move out of the way if the patient uses the legs to control the chair. The width, depth, and height of the chair must fit the patient's measurements. Patients must receive training in proper use of the chair, especially for safety considerations. There are a few innovative "high-tech" wheelchair designs that can rise up to bring the patient to a standing position and even climb stairs (the iBot and the Easycare Genie). Although both are expensive and more difficult to master, it is likely that technology-oriented baby boomers will use them more extensively.[29,30]

Many of the devices mentioned in the above pages are covered by Medicare Part B, with the potential for a 20% copayment, depending on whether the patient has secondary private insurance or Medicaid. **Table 1** illustrates coverage and useful sources of advice for some common items.

Power mobility devices include motorized wheelchairs and power-operated vehicles (POVs or scooters). They are somewhat controversial because of companies using illicit marketing techniques with elders in the community and Medicare fraud charges. Together they are labeled by the Centers for Medicare and Medicaid Services (CMS) as Mobility assistive equipment (MAE). CMS has produced a set of 9 questions the provider must answer to ensure Medicare coverage for an MAE (**Table 2**).[31] Some states require a rehabilitation specialist to evaluate the patient before CMS will cover the expense. Similar to an automobile, the patient must have the cognitive ability, finger control, and visual skills to operate such a vehicle. Ideally, the provider will conduct a safety "test drive" before the vehicle is finally released to the patient. Accidents and injuries with these chairs are fairly common, involving both the patients and others in the patient's living environment.

DEVICES FOR PATIENTS WHO WANDER

Wandering occurs in 15%–60% of people with dementia. Wandering can be beneficial, providing exercise and improving circulation. Subjects who wander generally enjoy better physical well-being and are able to maintain a balanced gait. On the other hand, wandering can be problematic to both people with dementia and their caregivers, causing physical harm and emotional distress and leading to earlier institutionalization. Hope and colleagues[32] reported that in a typical day, people with dementia and marked hyperactivity may walk all day without interruptions unless wandering is prevented.

In view of the harmful consequences associated with pharmacological methods and the ethical issues associated with the use of barrier/restraint methods to prevent wandering, a new perspective has evolved in the last decade with a shift from the prevention of wandering to the promotion of safe walking.[33] Alarms, locks, and

Table 1
Medicare coverage for commonly used assistive devices

Deficits	Potentially Useful Devices	Medicare Coverage	Team Member
Mobility	Canes: standard; four-prong Walkers: pickup; two-wheeled; front-wheeled; four-wheeled; Merry Walker (has seat) Self-propelled wheelchairs (leg rests, lightweight, and so on) Motorized wheelchairs, scooters	Standard cane (variable); four-prong (yes) Yes Yes Rigorous review, selective	PT
Dressing	Dressing sticks, buttonhooks, stocking gutters, long-handled shoehorns, reachers Clothing adaptations: grab loops on zippers; zippers that replace buttons; side-zip pants; sweats with long zippers; side-snap pants; back-flap pants; arm and leg protectors; footwear with Velcro closures; deep toe box shoe; plantar cushion; arch support	Yes Variable, often covered if provided during a rehabilitation unit stay.	OT
Eating	Plastic plate guards; rocker knives; two-handled spouted feeding cup; large-handled utensils; antisplash lids; angled silverware; steep-sided plates; non-slip mats; suction egg cups; lightweight insulated mugs	Yes	OT

Medication	Medication organizers ("pill box*"); electronic pager/timers; smart dispensers	No	RN
Bathroom	Portable devices: bath bench; rubber mat; hydraulic lift bath seats; bath stools or chairs; transfer bench; raised toilet seats Home adaptations: water thermostat; grab bars	Yes Device may be covered, installation not	OT, PT
Home Computers	Senior websites: http://www.seniornet.org, http://www.senior.com http://SeniorsForLiving.com Cell phone modifications: large backlit buttons; bright and large text; one-touch button feature; hearing-aid compatible PC modifications: voice recognition features; monitors with high-contrast, big display	No No No	OT

Abbreviations: OT, Occupational therapist; RN, Registered nurse.

Table 2
Medicare and Medicaid criteria for power wheelchair coverage
1. Does the beneficiary have a mobility limitation that significantly impairs his/her ability to participate in one or more MRADLs in the home?
2. Are there other conditions that limit the beneficiary's ability to participate in MRADLs at home?
3. If other limitations exist, can they be ameliorated or compensated sufficiently so that the MAE will be reasonably expected to significantly improve ability to perform or obtain assistance to participate in MRADLs in the home?
4. Does the beneficiary or caregiver demonstrate the capability and the willingness to consistently operate the MAE safely?
5. Can the functional mobility deficit be sufficiently resolved by a cane or walker?
6. Does the beneficiary's typical environment support the use of wheelchairs, including scooters/ POVs?
7. Does the beneficiary have sufficient upper-extremity function to propel a manual wheelchair in the home to participate in MRADLs during a typical day? The manual wheelchair should be optimally configured (seating options, wheelbase, device weight, and other appropriate accessories) for this determination.
8. Does the beneficiary have sufficient strength and postural stability to operate a POV/ scooter?
9. Are the additional features provided by a power wheelchair needed to allow the beneficiary to participate in one or more MRADLs?

Abbreviation: MRADLs, Mobility-related activities of daily living.

more sophisticated devices using blue tooth signals are among many interventions now in use.

Most typical wandering safety devices for the home emit an auditory signal to alert the caregiver. Door alerts can be simple and inexpensive electric sensors attached to door or optical sensors that generate an alarm when the person walks through. The drawback is that they cannot distinguish who is entering the monitored zone.

New technologies require the patient to wear a signal-transmitting device and can alert a caregiver through video call system. Some other antiwandering systems have the ability to lock peripheral doors and disable elevators. Motion detectors are infrared (IR) devices that allow caregivers to know if their elderly person is entering an area where they may be at risk. Sometimes they are linked to a lighting system that intensifies when the person enters the room. The dawn/dusk lights respond to ambient light levels. They are useful for elders who use the bathroom at night.

The Project Lifesaver program relies on radio technology and a specially trained search and rescue team. Clients who are enrolled in this program wear a personalized wristband that emits a tracking signal. When caregivers notify the local Lifesaver agency that the person is missing, a search and rescue team responds to the wanderer's area and starts searching with the mobile locater tracking system.

In general, non-pharmacological interventions are recommended to improve safety in wanderers, but there is limited evidence for their effectiveness, and they are not free from ethical concerns.[34]

DEVICES TO PROMOTE MEDICATION SAFETY AND ADHERENCE

Medication adherence is a key factor in remaining independent. Medication errors harm at least 1.5 million people every year in the United States.[35] Older adults consume 35% of all prescription drugs in the United States. It is estimated that between 40% and 60% of people do not take medication as prescribed, which can lead to worse health outcomes if the medications are needed and beneficial.

Medication devices (medication boxes) can increase patient compliance, as they help with remembering doses.[36] Metlay investigated the practices of community-dwelling adults taking high-risk medications. About 54% of participants indicated that they use a pillbox for organizing their medications. Of those who use pillboxes 92% use boxes with multiple compartments. The vast majority had boxes organized by week and filled the boxes themselves.[37] Currently, devices range from plastic boxes divided into sections labeled with time and dates to electronic systems that provide auditory cues and websites that help with scheduling medications.

Although they are widely available, only 2% of elders use "smart" medication dispensers, specifically a pillbox with an alarm. These electronic medication-dispensing units have several compartments for pills or other forms of medicine. During normal operation, the smart dispenser tracks the user's medication schedule, reminds the user when medications should be taken, controls the doses dispensed, and dynamically readjusts the medication schedule when the user is tardy. Some have a modem that can be set to call up to three phone numbers if a dose is missed. Heneghan's meta-analysis of medication-reminder systems indicated that they can increase the proportion of people taking their medications when measured by pill count.[36]

There are drawbacks to "smart" medication-reminder systems. Cost is one factor, with some devices priced as high as $800. Familiarity with device programming is essential; some home care nurses perform this function. Ideally, such systems will be linked to the physician's electronic medical record system, but few have this capability.

DEVICES FOR FIRE SAFETY

Each year, approximately 1,100 Americans aged 65 and older die as a result of a home fire. Compared to the rest of the US population, elders older than 75 years are nearly four times as likely to die in a fire. Although careless smoking and cooking are leading causes of fire-related injury among elderly people, faulty or misused electrical items, particularly electric blankets, cause the most fatalities.[38] The home environment can be modified to reduce injuries and deaths from fires. Modifications include smoke and fire alarms, sprinkler systems, fire extinguishers, and devices such as rope ladders.

Fire alarms are recommended for elders who smoke or cook at home and are at increased risk of causing a fire. They work by measuring the absolute temperature and rate of change of temperature. Smoke alarms react to visible and invisible fire aerosols by using an optical or ionization detector. Therefore, they can detect a fire at an earlier stage than a fire alarm. Peek-Asa[39] estimated that residents of homes without a smoke alarm have 3.4 times the risk of fire death as residents of homes with a smoke alarm.[40] Hall reported that smoke detectors cut the risk of dying in a home fire by about 40%.[41]

Elders with hearing loss and those on multiple medications may not hear the standard 55–75 dB alarm usually installed in a hallway. Therefore, it is recommended that smoke detector alarms be installed in the bedrooms and that the signal intensity should be 90 dB, the maximum level tolerable to the human ear.[41] Although smoke alarms are highly effective, their use is not universal after nearly 3 decades of availability. Approximately 88% of homes have at least one installed smoke alarm, but one-quarter to one-third of alarms are nonfunctional. Reported explanations are difficulties with alarm maintenance plus stress created by false alarms.[42] DiGuiseppi and Higgins' review on smoke alarm ownership concluded that educational programs that promote smoke alarm installation and maintenance had modest effects on increasing smoke alarm ownership or functionality.[43] The role of home sprinkler systems in saving lives has not been documented. Although sprinklers would require very little maintenance, the ability of owners to manage complex sprinkler systems is not known and may be poor, as suggested by the lack of maintenance of smoke alarms.

HOME COMPUTERS AS ASSISTIVE DEVICES

The US Census Bureau reported that about 34% of elders go online regularly. Usage decreases to 28% for those aged 70 years and older. When compared with seniors, Internet usage by other age groups is "near universal."[44] Of the 12 million seniors who go online 68% (8.1 million) use the Internet to locate health information.[45] Differences in computer use can be a consequence of aging itself, such as decline in vision, hearing, and manual dexterity; but there is also a generational effect, because personal computer (PC) use has only been widespread for 20 years. Currently, there are many services aiming to bridge the "gray" digital gap. Computers can be found in every public library and most senior centers. National educational networks that teach older adults computer skills are growing fast. For example, many public libraries have programs dedicated to training seniors in the use of the Internet.[46]

Online services can be helpful when disabled and homebound, affording the ability to perform tasks the person may have been unable to execute without personal help, such as managing finances through online banking, ordering supermarket goods, and keeping current by reading online newspapers, magazines, and books. Going online also provides social contacts and networking. Some seniors use PCs to locate health care information. The typical Internet-enabled senior is female, white, has postgraduate education and higher income, and owns a computer.

Whether they are looking for information about health problems or looking up vacation options, sending an e-mail to a grandchild, or discussing politics with friends in an online chat room, older adults are taking advantage of the Internet. Today, we can find seniors everywhere we go online, but many gather in SeniorNet (http://www.seniornet. org), the largest, most popular senior-related web network. Offering online computer training, senior events, and membership applications, plus a busy chat room, this popular site is a sort of virtual community for the aged to talk about current issues and the good old times. A World War II forum has attracted much attention from veterans in search of wartime companions and school-age users who like to question older members about their experiences growing up and living through the war.

Another popular online site for elders is Senior.com (http://www.senior.com). This site provides a comprehensive starting point from which older adults may connect to other senior-related sites. The site offers easy access to information about government programs, health and fitness, volunteer opportunities, financial and legal services, links to travel sites, a Free Store that links to complimentary services and products on the Internet, and a virtual newsstand with online editions of popular magazines, newspapers, and books. A new path to tracking current events and meeting people from around the world is through blogging. In SeniorsForLiving.com there is information about 100 senior blogs and retiree housing Internet destinations.

Many hardware and software innovations are available for people with disabilities. Computer manufacturers are building devices with adaptations to better accommodate people with hearing, visual, and physical impairments. For example, Windows lets users with physical handicaps configure the keyboard and mouse for easier execution of keyboard- and click commands. It lets hearing-impaired users substitute visual signals for audio signals, and visually impaired users can set the monitor for a high-contrast, easily visible display. There are touch-pads that require little wrist motion and voice recognition allows users eliminate the keyboard and mouse altogether. Alternative forms of data entry, such as IR pointing devices maneuvered by head movement or sip-and-puff switches controlled by breathing techniques, provide users with multiple impairments the chance to do things for themselves.

Cell phone technology is also changing to meet elders' needs. Some companies offer a wide variety of senior plans and packages. Simple, larger backlit buttons and bright, large text are available. Most phones are hearing aid compatible. Newer speaker sounds are louder and clearer. Special service includes 24-hour operators who can make calls for the elder with the use of a one-touch button feature. More interesting, a Motorola cell phone can determine that the user is older through speech acoustics based upon lower speech rate, less energy, and trembling within the speech utterances. Once recognized, the cell phone adjusts incoming audio by boosting the high-frequency bands through audio processors while simultaneously increasing the power of the outgoing signal to improve intelligibility. Additionally, the graphical user interface is automatically changed to adjust based on the visual characteristics of elderly users. Font size is increased and menu structures are simplified, making the phone easier to use.

SMART HOME TECHNOLOGY

SHs can be defined as a system of "information and communication technology in homes where components communicate through a local network."[47] Home automation systems are being developed in two basic forms - embedded health systems and private health networks. Embedded Health Systems involve use of sensors and microprocessors located within in appliances, furniture, and clothing, which collect data that can be analyzed and used for a variety of purposes, such as detecting physiologic changes. These systems are still experimental and are not generally available. Private health networks use wireless and wired technology to connect devices in the home and allow for others (such as caregivers) to monitor a homebound elder. These types of systems are becoming more common and affordable.

SH technology has been available since the 1980s but the advent of the Internet and PC have greatly expanded the opportunities. The BESTA project in Norway has been using SH technology since 1994 in patient's homes. Though many programs have been implemented in Europe, few studies have tested the effectiveness of SH technology. One randomized trial of the effect of the use of SH technology by frail elders[48] using X-10 devices (discussed below) revealed that the treatment group participants maintained physical and cognitive status, whereas the control group declined. After 2 years, 80% of the treatment group remained in their homes compared with 66% of controls. The cost of the devices averaged only $400, excluding the PC. However, the cost of installing the devices was not measured. Satisfaction was high, and 91% would recommend the system to others.

Many purposes can be served through SH technology, including enhancing safety, increasing access to care providers, providing off-site and asynchronous monitoring of activities, and promoting independence. Although there are a number of experimental SHs in academic medical settings, such as the University of Florida (Gator-Tech Smart Home [GTSH]), fewer systems have been fully implemented in individual's homes. This section describes a fully implemented version of SH technology located in an assisted living facility, Oatfield Estates in Milwaukie, OR.[49] The hardware and software applications are exportable to a home setting.

Each resident at Oatfield Estates has a PC in their room with an elder-friendly interface that has large fonts and icons and touch screen capability. The in-room computer is connected via the Internet to a central server in administration. Photos of caregivers are prominently displayed, and a simple touch of the picture sends a radio frequency (RF) signal to the caregiver that help is needed. The rooms are fitted with a number of off-the-shelf transmitters that are designed to control door locks, lighting, room temperature, and ceiling fans. Load sensors beneath beds determine when the resident is in bed and measure their weight. Residents wear on their shirt or blouse a transmitter that is equipped for both IR and RF transmission.

Based on an assessment by a trained care provider (such as a nurse), the resident's personal care program is programmed into the database. This allows a wide variety of SH-based interventions tailored to the resident's needs. For instance, if a resident awakens at night frequently to go to the bathroom, the load cells on the bed will detect the resident getting out of bed. The system can be programmed to turn on the lights in the bathroom. Similarly, persons with memory deficits may have problems remembering their room or the use of a key. Locks can be programmed to open automatically when the door sensor detects proximity of the resident to his or her own room.

When a resident calls for a caregiver (there are multiple options for calling, including touching the caregiver picture icon on the PC, touching the shirt pendant, or a pull-cord in the room or bathroom), the caregiver receives notification on a Wi–Fi-equipped personal digital assistant (PDA). All resident's door locks are programmed to unlock when the caregiver is in close proximity. The time of the call for assistance, the caregiver's reading of the call, the arrival at the door, and the time spent in the room are all recorded by the program. The caregiver then attends to the resident's needs and documents the intervention in the PDA. The data from these interactions can be used for many purposes: to ensure quality of care, to provide feedback to employees on their performance, to assure regulators, surveyors, accrediting agencies, and family members that the resident's needs have been addressed, and to inform caregivers of need to modify care plans.

One major concern with SH technology is cost. Many builders are building new homes with all rooms wired for Internet, and wireless systems have also greatly reduced costs. One of the most cost-effective methods for upgrading existing homes is the X-10 system. This system was invented in Scotland in 1975 and uses the house's electrical wiring to send digital data between modules that attach to various household devices (such as lights, garage door openers, or kitchen equipment) and a combination of PC and RF devices to control the equipment. It is relatively inexpensive and easily available from a variety of Internet vendors. Products include such devices as light controls, door and window sensors, motion sensors, chimes for reminding people to turn off the stove or take medications, and video capabilities for viewing the property or guests at the front door (or the resident within the house). Control units can be freestanding or operated through a PC.

SH systems can be integrated with other assistive devices. For instance, reminder systems can be programmed to provide a verbal cue to take medications, wash hands, or turn off appliances. Fall protection systems can be linked to automatically dial for help, and some central control units have loud speakers and sensitive microphones that can detect a person's voice throughout the house. The GTSH includes pressure sensors in the floors that can detect if a person falls, or remains motionless for a prolonged time, and notify the caregiver. If a PC is used as the controller, the calendar program can be directed to verbally remind the client of an appointment.

There are numerous concerns about SH technology. As with all assistive devices, the patient must be adequately assessed for need, trained in device use, and capable and motivated to use them. Unfortunately, many of the current interfaces are not designed with older people in mind. Internet sites for device purchase are often difficult to read and negotiate. Though the devices themselves are relatively inexpensive, installation can be costly. Perhaps the most challenging aspect is concerns about potential intrusiveness of some applications and ethical issues surrounding their use. This is particularly true regarding observations of the patient's living space by others such as family members or caregivers.

Fear of "Big Brother" looking over every aspect of a homebound elder life is natural. However, as noted above, older users have generally favorable attitudes toward SH technology. In addition, in a study using focus groups, Johnson and colleagues[50] found that all participants without significant functional impairment thought remote monitoring was a good idea, but not for them at this time. Of those with impairments, there was a range of attitudes, with many not wanting it. These findings emphasize the importance of informed consent and collaborative decision making when considering SH technology. Older persons must balance the threat of loss of independent living with the perceived burdens of the use of any AT.

SUMMARY

AT can enable older adults to remain in the home for longer periods and avoid institutionalization. All assistive devices have both benefits and burdens. The most important aspect of providing an assistive device is proper assessment to determine the "person-device fit." Every device, from a simple bath aid to SH technology, has the risk of not being used, or worse, injuring the older adult, if it is not correctly prescribed, the patient is poorly trained in its use, or the patient does not desire it.

REFERENCES

1. Federal interagency forum on aging-related statistics. Older Americans 2008: key indicators of well-being. Available at: http://www.agingstats.gov/agingstatsdotnet/Main_Site/Data/2008_Documents/Health_Status.aspx. Accessed July 23, 2008.
2. Administration on aging, statistical data on the aging. Available at: http://www.aoa.gov/prof/statistics/online_stat_data/online_stat_data.aspx. Accessed July 13, 2008.
3. Marek KD, Popejoy L, Petroski G, et al. Clinical outcomes of aging in place. Nurs Res 2005;54:202–11.
4. Russell JN, Hendershot GE, LeClere F, et al. Trends and differential use of assistive technology devices: United States, 1994. Washington DC: National Center for Health Statistics; 1997.
5. Hoenig H. Assistive technology and mobility aids for the older patient with disability. Ann Long Term Care 2004;12:12–9.
6. Assistive Technology Act of 1998. Available at: http://www.ed.gov/policy/speced/guid/rsa/tac-06-02.doc. Accessed July 23, 2008.
7. Available at: www.abledata.com. Accessed July 19, 2008.
8. Kitchener M, Ng T, Lee HY, et al. Assistive technology in Medicaid home- and community-based waiver programs. Gerontologist 2008;48:181–9.
9. Manton KG. Recent declines in chronic disability in the elderly U.S. Population: risk factors and future dynamics. Annu Rev Public Health 2008;29:91–113.

10. Agree EM, Freedman VA. Incorporating assistive devices into community-based long-term care: an analysis of the potential for substitution and supplementation. J Aging Health 2000;12:426–50.
11. Freedman VA, Martin LG, Schoeni RF. Recent trends in disability and functioning among older adults in the United States: a systematic review. J Am Med Assoc 2002;288:3137–46.
12. Agree EM, Freedman VA. A comparison of assistive technology and personal care in alleviating disability and unmet need. Gerontologist 2003;43:335–44.
13. Taylor DH, Hoenig H. The effect of equipment usage and residual task difficulty on use of personal assistance, days in bed, and nursing home placement. J Am Geriatr Soc 2004;52:72–9.
14. Verbrugge LM, Rennert C, Madans JH. The great efficacy of personal and equipment assistance in reducing disability. Am J Public Health 1997;87:384–92.
15. Verbrugge L, Sevak P. Use, type, and efficacy of assistance for disability. J Gerontol B Psychol Sci Soc Sci 2002;57(6):S366–79.
16. Mann WC, Ottenbacher K, Fraas L, et al. Effectiveness of assistive technology and environmental interventions in maintaining independence and reducing home care costs for the frail elderly: a randomized trial. Arch Fam Med 1999;8: 210–7.
17. Kraskowsky L, Finlayson M. Factors affecting older adults' use of adaptive equipment: review of the literature. Am J Occup Ther 2001;55:303–10.
18. Available at: http://www.ap.buffalo.edu/idea/Home/index.asp. Accessed July 31, 2008.
19. Available at: http://design.ncsu.edu/cud. Accessed July 31, 2008.
20. Hoenig H, Piper C, Zolkewitz M, et al. Wheelchair users are not necessarily wheelchair bound. J Am Geriatr Soc 2002;50:645–54.
21. Amella EJ. Assessment and management of eating and feeding difficulties for older people. Geriatr Nurs 1998;19:269–75.
22. Connolly MJ, Wilson AS. Feeding aids. BMJ 1990;301:378–9.
23. Hobbs FB, Damon BL. 65 + in the United States. Washington, DC: U.S. Government Printing Office; 1996.
24. Mann WC, Kimble C, Justiss MD, et al. Problems with dressing in the frail elderly. Am J Occup Ther 2005;59:398–408.
25. Mann WC, Hurren D, Tomita M, et al. Use of assistive devices for bathing by elderly who are not institutionalized. Occup Ther J Res 1996;16:261–86.
26. Gill TM, Han L, Allore HG. Bath aids and the subsequent development of bathing disability in community-living older persons. J Am Geriatr Soc 2007;55:1757–63.
27. Murphy S, Gretebeck KA, Alexander NB. The bath environment, the bathing task, and the older adult: a review and future directions for bathing disability research. Disabil Rehabil 2007;29:1067–75.
28. Constantinescu R, Leonard C, Deeley C, et al. Assistive devices for gait in Parkinson's disease. Parkinsonism Relat Disord 2007;13:133–8.
29. Available at: http://www.ibotnow.com/. Accessed July 31, 2008.
30. Available at: http://www.onhealthcare.ie/onhealthcare/Main/Wheelchairs_Easy care_Genie.htm. Accessed July 31, 2008.
31. Available at: http://www.cms.hhs.gov/mlnproducts/downloads/pmdfactsheet07_quark19.pdf. Accessed July 31, 2008.
32. Hope T, Keene J, McShane RH, et al. Wandering in dementia: a longitudinal study. Int Psychogeriatr 2001;13:137–47.
33. Robinson L, Hutchings D, Corner L, et al. A systematic literature review of the effectiveness of non-pharmacological interventions to prevent wandering in

dementia and evaluation of the ethical implications and acceptability of their use. Health Technol Assess 2006;10:1–126.
34. Hermans DG, Htay UHla McShane R. Non-pharmacological interventions for wandering of people with dementia in the domestic setting. Cochrane Database Syst Rev 2007, Issue 1. Art. No.: CD005994. DOI 10.1002/14651858.CD005994.pub2.
35. Aspden P, Wolcott JA, Bootman L, et al. Committee on Identifying and Preventing Medication Errors and the Board on Health Care Services. Preventing Medication Errors (Quality Chasm Series). Washington, DC, National Academies Press 2007;357:624–25.
36. Heneghan CJ, Glasziou PP, Perera R. Reminder packaging for improving adherence to self-administered long-term medications. Cochrane Database Syst Rev 2006:CD005025.
37. Metlay JP, Cohen A, Polsky D, et al. Medication safety in older adults: home-based practice patterns. J Am Geriatr Soc 2005;53:976–82.
38. Elder AT, Squires T, Busuttil A. Fire fatalities in elderly people. Age Ageing 1996; 25:214–6.
39. Peek-Asa C, Zwerling C. Role of environmental interventions in injury control and prevention. Epidemiol Rev 2003;25:77–89.
40. Hall JR Jr. The U.S. experience with smoke detectors: who has them? How well do they work? When don't they work? NFPA J 1994;88:36–46.
41. Bruck D. The who, what, where and why of waking to fire alarms: a review. Fire Saf J 2001;36:623–39.
42. Roberts J, Curtis K, Liabo K, et al. Putting public health evidence into practice: increasing the prevalence of working smoke alarms in disadvantaged inner city housing. Epidemiol Community Health 2004;58:280–5.
43. DiGuiseppi C, Higgins JPT. Interventions for promoting smoke alarm ownership and function (Cochrane Review). The Cochrane Library, issue 2. Oxford: United Kingdom Update Software Ltd; 2002.
44. Fox S. Online health search 2006. Pew Internet & American life project. Available at: http://www.pewinternet.org/PPF/r/190/report_display.asp. Accesses July 5, 2008.
45. Campbell RJ. Meeting seniors' information needs: using computer technology. Home Health Care Manag Pract 2008;20:328–35.
46. Web savvy seniors: Internet training for seniors at the public library. Available at: http://www.slais.ubc.ca/COURSES/libr500/04-05-wt2/www/M_Sanders/introduction.htm. Accessed July 23, 2008.
47. Cheek P. Aging well with smart technology. Nurs Adm Q 2005;29:329–38.
48. Tomita MR, Mann WC, Statnton K, et al. Use of currently available smart home technology by frail elders. Top Geriatr Rehabil 2007;23:24–34.
49. Available at: http://www.elitecare.com/oatfield_estates. Accessed July 19, 2008.
50. Johnson JL, Davenport R, Mann WC. Consumer feedback on smart home applications. Top Geriatr Rehabil 2007;23:60–72.

Hospital at Home

Jennifer Cheng, MD[a], Michael Montalto, MBBS, PhD[b,c,d], Bruce Leff, MD[e,*]

KEYWORDS

• Home health care • Hospital at home • House calls

In 2006, national health expenditures in the United States of $2.1 trillion represented 16% of the gross domestic product. Of that, 31% was spent on acute hospital care, with Medicare paying the hospital bill for nearly 30%.[1] Despite these massive and ever increasing expenditures, a number of reports, including the seminal "To Err is Human, Building a Safer Health Care System" from the Institute of Medicine (IOM), highlight the fact that health care quality and patient safety are a significant concern during acute hospital care.[2,3]

Iatrogenic events occur commonly in acute care hospitals. The Harvard Medical Practice Studies found that approximately 4% of hospitalized patients suffered an adverse event; more than two-thirds of these were due to errors. These events were more common among older patients, even after adjustment for comorbid medical conditions.[4–6] Using these and other data, the IOM estimated that at least 44,000 people die in US hospitals each year due to medical mistakes at a cost between $37 and $50 billion. Many studies suggest that the elderly are at especially high risk and frequently experience adverse events, such as functional decline, pressure sores, nosocomial infections, and delirium.[7–9] In addition, preventable adverse events also occur during the transition from hospital to home at hospital discharge, the result of deficiencies in health system design and poor communication.[10,11]

Other secular trends favor alternatives to traditional acute hospital care. These include expectation of patients as consumers of health services for more personalized and safer care;[12,13] creation of safe, portable, advanced hospital-type technologies; equally rapid development in domestic technologies that enhance information transfer and personal care; access to hospitalization for an increasing number and range of interventions; and attempts by funders of health care to examine alternatives to traditional hospitalization.

[a] Johns Hopkins Bayview Medical Center, 4940 Eastern Avenue, Johns Hopkins University School of Medicine, Baltimore, MD 21224, USA
[b] Hospital in the Home, 89 Bridge Road, Richmond, Victoria 3121, Australia
[c] Epworth Hospital, 89 Bridge Road, Richmond, Victoria 3121, Australia
[d] Royal Melbourne Hospital, Melbourne, Victoria, Australia
[e] Division of Geriatric Medicine and Gerontology, Department of Medicine, Johns Hopkins University School of Medicine, Johns Hopkins Bayview Medical Center, 5505 Hopkins Bayview Circle, Baltimore, MD 21224, USA
* Corresponding author.
E-mail address: bleff@jhmi.edu (B. Leff).

Clin Geriatr Med 25 (2009) 79–91
doi:10.1016/j.cger.2008.10.002
0749-0690/08/$ – see front matter © 2009 Elsevier Inc. All rights reserved.

geriatric.theclinics.com

Improving the quality and safety of care in acute care hospitals is critically important, as hospitals are an essential component of the health care system. However, as the population continues to age and grow frail, and as hospitals evolve into the setting for the delivery of increasingly high-technology critical care, developing alternative systems to provide treatment of acute medical illness is vital.

Hospital at home (HaH) is one such alternative. HaH is generally defined as the clinical activity that administers therapy and technology usually associated with acute inpatient care, but in a community setting. HaH patients are those who, without the provision of the HaH service, would require inpatient care.

In this article, we define the HaH model of care and describe the scope of HaH in terms of the types of health conditions and patients that can be treated and the role of the HaH physician. We then review the evidence base on the outcomes of HaH and describe the dissemination of the HaH model into widespread practice. Finally, we discuss recent advances in the related issue of high-tech home care.

DEFINING HOSPITAL AT HOME CARE

Clearly defining a health service delivery intervention has been too often overlooked in the measurement and development of effective or innovative health services. Defining a service clearly can be especially difficult when dealing with a new service whose properties may be in dispute or in evolution. HaH is one such example.

A variety of care models have been included under the broad HaH definition, including programs that substitute entirely for an inpatient hospital admission and, more commonly, those that facilitate early discharge from the acute care hospital. Some programs have focused solely on patients following surgery, while others have targeted patients with medical conditions. Nurses deliver the bulk of care in most models; few have included substantial physician presence. Some models have focused on distinct populations, such as children. The wide variety of models claiming HaH status probably reflects the fact that most published models developed in countries with national health care systems in which the HaH model fills a particular clinical niche.

There are 4 main types of HaH models documented in the literature. The first is the outpatient infusion center where patients receive an intravenous infusion or other treatment.[14] Next is the physicians' office intravenous infusion service where patients usually self-infuse their medications and are supervised in physicians' offices.[15–17] The third type is at-home delivery by hospital, hospital contracted staff, or, in the United States, by a home health agency of care, mostly for surgical patients, in which patients are sent home early in the postoperative period and receive postoperative nursing supervision and skilled therapies at home with little or no organized input from physicians.[18–29] The final model is a substitutive HaH that delivers acute hospital-level care in a patient's home in lieu of acute hospital admission—in these models nursing care is always provided, and physician inputs are often available but have been variably used.[30–41]

This variety of models has engendered controversy over the definition of HaH as well as the perceived overall effectiveness of the concept.[42,43] The Cochrane Collaboration Review of HaH[44] includes articles on models that have little in common with each other and little adherence to a common set of underlying principles, other than that the disparate services provide "active treatment by health care professions, in the patient's home, of a condition that would require acute hospital inpatient care, always for a limited period."

We suggest that the HaH model most likely to be associated with successful outcomes for patients and health systems is a "clinical unit" model characterized by 1) treatment at home of an acute condition of a severity that normally requires hospitalization; 2) treatment that requires hospital-type technologies or hospital-level care; 3) acceptance of responsibility by the hospital or health system for the acute care episode, and HaH patients retain inpatient status; 4) funding, provision of pharmaceuticals, pathology, radiology, and other services, which are delivered according to standards commensurate with inpatient status and appropriate to the patient's level of medical acuity; 5) physician care at home, provided by identified HaH doctors with 24-hour coverage; 6) direct nursing care, provided at home with 24-hour coverage; 7) care that is provided in a coordinated manner similar to that in an inpatient hospital ward; and 8) consent to treatment by patients. Thus defined, HaH functions as a distinct but integrated ward of a hospital, albeit without the usual bricks and mortar. The HaH accepts direct admissions from the emergency department or ambulatory site for "substitutive HaH," which substitutes entirely for acute hospital admission. HaH can also accept transfers from other inpatient services for patients who continue to require inpatient-level care in the same manner that in-hospital transfers between ward may occur, for example, from the intensive care unit to a medical ward.

This is distinct from "early discharge" or "facilitated discharge" programs, which constitute the bulk of the literature and provide community-based home care without much physician presence. These have value but should be distinguished from HaH. Defining HaH in this manner satisfies the underlying rationale for the model described here to the greatest extent. In discussing outcomes, we review evidence related to the substitutive HaH construct described in the preceding paragraph.

SCOPE OF HAH: CONDITIONS, PATIENTS, TREATMENTS, AND THE PHYSICIAN'S ROLE

Table 1 offers examples of the wide range of conditions that can be or have been treated with HaH. Patients tend to have these characteristics in common: 1) the condition occurs frequently and accounts for a significant portion of hospitalizations; 2) the diagnosis is relatively uncomplicated and can thus be made rapidly without much consultation or invasive testing; and 3) the treatment is well defined and can be delivered in a feasible, safe, and efficient manner at home.[45] Substitutive HaH models have addressed heart failure, chronic obstructive airway disease, bronchiectasis, community-acquired pneumonia, urinary tract infection, cellulitis, exacerbations of Parkinson's disease and multiple sclerosis, diarrhea and vomiting, first ischemic stroke, minor strokes, venous thromboembolism, and infections requiring intravenous antibiotics, such as endocarditis and osteomyelitis.

HaH programs have focused mainly on older patients, identifying potential patients by diagnosis and morbidity risk. With rare exceptions, few have described stringent selection criteria other than rejecting patients who need intensive care. Most have required that patients have caregivers available. A few programs have accepted patients from nursing homes. All describe the need to operate in a limited geographic area to enable timely response to urgent clinical situations. There are few data to characterize patients who chose HaH over facility-based care. Unpublished data from a US study suggest that there are few sociodemographic or health status differences between these 2 groups, and the decision to choose HaH is based on preferences. Those who believe that home-based treatment is associated with greater "comfort and convenience" tend to choose HaH care. Patients who believe that they would be "safer in the hospital," tend to choose traditional acute hospital care.

Table 1 Examples of conditions treated in hospital at home	
Infectious diseases	• Community-acquired pneumonia • Bronchiectasis • Infective exacerbations of other chronic airways disease • Skin, bursal, and soft-tissue infections • Urinary tract infections • Bone and joint infections • Endocarditis • Prosthesis-related infections of all types • Hospital-acquired and other multiresistant infections • Febrile neutropenia • Cytomegalovirus retinitis • Herpes simplex
Dehydration and Volume Depletion	• Mild dehydration in elderly due to gastroenteritis • Hyperemesis of pregnancy
Venous Thromboembolic Disease	• Acute deep venous thrombosis • Pulmonary embolism
Cardiac Disease	• Heart failure • Atrial fibrillation
Miscellaneous	• Ischemic cerebrovascular accident • Multiple sclerosis • Ulcerative colitis • Decompensated liver disease • Parkinson's disease

Table 2 describes examples of therapies that have been deployed in HaH models. With continued advancement of health care technologies, including telehealth monitoring and medical therapies, both the types of medical conditions and patient population managed by HaH are expected to expand.

The physician's role in HaH has varied widely. As noted, early discharge models at best involve physicians in supervision at a distance; substitutive HaH models also report varied physician roles. In some models, community-based general practitioners are available for home visits to HaH patients but make few visits. Other models require that physicians visit the patients at home every day on the premise that HaH patients require the same care that they would have received inside hospital walls. There appears to be a relationship between clinical benefits obtained and the degree of physician participation in providing HaH care.

OUTCOMES OF HOSPITAL AT HOME

A range of clinical outcomes have been reported in HaH studies, including complications, quality of care provided, quality of life, patient and caregiver satisfaction with care, caregiver stress, functional autonomy, survival, and use and cost of health services. We focus on outcomes of early discharge and substitutive models, as labeled and reported in the literature. In these studies, HaH care is compared with traditional acute hospital care with the expectation that HaH clinical outcomes should

Table 2
Examples of therapies delivered by hospital at home (HoH)
Intravenous Antibiotic Therapy for the Treatment of a Variety of Infectious Diseases
Intravenous corticosteroids
Intravenous fluid therapy
Intravenous antiviral therapy
Acute anticoagulation therapy
Intravenous inotropic and diuretic therapy
Intravenous blood product infusion
Intravenous chemotherapy
Oxygen therapy
Simple radiology, eg, chest and abdominal radiographs, ultrasound, venous Doppler, and cardiac echocardiography
Procedures such as paracentesis and thoracentesis

be at least equivalent if not superior to outcomes associated with acute hospital care, and at least cost neutral.

An IOM[46] report on outcomes from HaH care for multi-morbid older people divided studies into "early discharge" and "substitutive" categories; some models had both components. Nine randomized controlled trials of early discharge models were included.[20,21,24–29,47,48] These typically did not require physician home visits and provided services that, in the United States, would be called skilled home care. Three studies focused on chronic obstructive pulmonary disease[27–29] and 2 on stroke rehabilitation.[24,25] While all studies examined use and costs of health services, 8 assessed survival, 5 assessed functional outcomes, 5 assessed quality of life, and none assessed quality of care. Three studies included measures for patient satisfaction and showed increased satisfaction,[21,24,48] but only 2 demonstrated statistical significance. Impact on length of stay was variable, 1 cost-minimization analysis showed lower cost,[48] and 1 found no cost difference.[21] Early discharge models generally showed no difference in quality of life, functional autonomy, and survival compared to traditional hospitalization; 1 study reported increased quality of life and instrumental activities of daily living (IADL) function.[47] Possible explanations for the equivocal findings include diverse patient populations and treatments; minimal physician involvement; varied sample size; and limited outcome data.

Studies of substitutive HaH models also included varied models, target populations, and outcomes. Compared with early discharge models, substitutive models demonstrated better outcomes across a range of categories. We review several of these programs in detail.

The Jerusalem, Israel, HaH program[49] had both early discharge and substitutive elements and was evaluated in a quasi-experimental study. This model accepted patients older than 65 years either to in-home, physician-supervised interdisciplinary medical care or to usual care. Annual hospitalization per enrollee decreased compared with utilization the year before the study and compared with hospitalization in the control group. The program avoided 8,486 hospital days during the 26-month study, providing substantial savings for the managed care-type plan that deployed the model. Patient satisfaction was high.

In the Leicester, UK, HaH, Wilson and colleagues randomly assigned 199 patients to admission-avoidance HaH care or traditional hospital care. General practitioners provided medical coverage, but they were minimally involved; home care was provided by nurses. Intention-to-treat analyses found significantly shorter length of stay for the HaH group than that for the hospital group (8 versus 14.5 days). There were no differences in emergency department visits after discharge from the index admission, mortality, functional status, or quality of life.[38] Cost-minimization analysis found significantly lower cost in the HaH group.[39] There was increased patient and caregiver satisfaction, assessed by the Caregiver Strain Index and semi-structured interviews. Reasons for greater satisfaction included more personal care, better communication, and therapeutic benefits of staying at home. Patients felt safe in HaH, though some would have felt safer in hospital. Caregivers felt the workload imposed by patients staying at home is no greater than traditional hospitalization.[50]

In an Australian randomized controlled trial, Caplan and colleagues[30] studied 100 patients who had caregivers and met criteria for acute hospitalization randomly assigned to HaH or usual hospitalization. Patients had varied conditions including pneumonia and heart failure. Physicians were available but on average made only 1 home visit during the acute admission in the home. This study notably showed that HaH care was associated with significantly fewer geriatric complications, all with single-digit "numbers needed to prevent" an adverse outcome. These geriatric complications, assessed by medical record review, were confusion, urinary complications, constipation, and fecal incontinence. There were higher levels of satisfaction among patients and caregivers and improvements in the ability to perform IADLs.[40] There were no differences in mortality or hospital readmission rates. Costs were significantly lower in the HaH group.[41]

Several disease-specific studies from Italy have demonstrated excellent results. In a randomized trial of HaH for elderly patients with advanced dementia requiring acute hospitalization, Tibaldi and colleagues[33] reported significant reductions in behavioral disturbance among HaH patients, with no difference in mortality. Administration of antipsychotic medications was reduced, and caregiver stress was lower. It is likely that these benefits were related to preserving familiar environments and routines for these severely demented individuals. Reporting on a randomized controlled trial of 120 patients with first acute ischemic stroke, Ricauda and colleagues[32] found no difference in patient satisfaction with HaH in the same Italian program; HaH patients did experience greater improvement in depression scores and were more likely to remain at home rather than being admitted to nursing home at 6 months.[34] Cost-minimization analysis revealed savings. Finally, in a randomized trial of HaH for patients with chronic obstructive pulmonary disease, Ricauda and colleagues[31] demonstrated greater improvement in depression scores, better quality-of-life scores, lower costs, and lower rates of readmission to hospital at 6 months (42% versus 87%). An important advantage of this program compared with other HaH models is relative maturity. Most HaH studies are of newly implemented models, due to the need for demonstrating the financial value of a novel and relatively expensive clinical service to justify maintaining its operation.

At Johns Hopkins University, Leff and colleagues[45] have developed substitutive HaH with a robust physician component. Initially, several acute medical conditions that were appropriate for HaH care were identified, and medical eligibility criteria were validated to select appropriate HaH patients. The identified conditions were community-acquired pneumonia, chronic heart failure, chronic obstructive pulmonary disease, and cellulitis. Pilot studies demonstrated clinical and economic feasibility.[51] Because HaH does not fit traditional Medicare fee-for-service payment well, larger studies were performed in integrated health care delivery systems, such as Medicare managed care and the Veterans Affairs health systems. The Hopkins model employs initial continuous nursing care, followed by intermittent nurse visits, and at least daily physician home visits. A randomized controlled trial was forbidden by the Center for Medicare and Medicaid services because of regulations governing Medicare managed-care plans. Using a quasi-experimental design with a conservative intent-to-treat analysis, HaH care was shown to be feasible and efficacious. Patients received timely hospital-level care at home that met quality standards.[37] Compared with patients treated in the acute hospital, those treated in HaH suffered fewer important clinical complications, including sedative medication use, chemical restraints, and incident delirium. Patient and family member satisfaction was higher.[36] Although patients were not required to have a caregiver (30% lived alone), caregiver stress was lower.[35] HaH patients improved in the ability to perform IADLs compared with usual care patients.[52] The average amount paid for HaH patients was lower; savings resulted from reduced use of laboratory and high-tech procedures.[53]

Overall, the literature suggests that HaH is feasible and efficacious. Substitutive models that target patients appropriately and provide substantial physician input appear to produce better outcomes than early discharge models with scant physician input.

DISSEMINATION OF HAH INTO WIDESPREAD PRACTICE

In a popular theory of diffusion of innovations, Rogers[54] identified 3 clusters of influence on dissemination: perceptions of the innovation, characteristics of potential adopters of an innovation, and contextual factors, such as communication, incentives, and leadership. Regarding perceptions of the innovation, 5 factors are theorized to be critical: 1) relative advantages compared with current practice; 2) compatibility with values, beliefs, and needs of potential adopters; 3) complexity; 4) whether the innovation can be tested easily before a significant investment in adoption is made ("trialability"); and 5) observability, the ease with which a potential adopter can observe others try the innovation first. Generally, innovations that have significant relative advantage, are compatible with existing systems and culture, are simple, are trialable, and are observable are more likely to be successfully diffused in what is envisioned as a passive, unplanned, informal, and decentralized process.

While clear clinical advantages have been demonstrated for HaH, it is a complex model[55] and thus faces dissemination barriers. HaH models have not been described in sufficient detail in the literature to allow potential adopters to understand all relevant adoption issues. The evidence base focuses on patient-related outcomes to the relative exclusion of other outcomes relevant to potential adopters. As a complex model, HaH may clash with a potential adopting organization's prevailing culture. HaH is not easily trialable since it requires a specialized team, making it difficult to pull "off the shelf." HaH requires collaboration among stakeholders within and, at times, between organizations, and the entire model must be developed before the first patient can be enrolled. Finally, there are few HaH units extant to observe the model in action.

However, in the United States, the most important barrier is that the business case for adoption is constrained by current fee-for-service payment. Under Medicare payment, a hospital or health system has no incentive to deploy HaH. To do so would require expending resources while losing revenue that would come from usual care hospital admission. Integrated delivery systems, such as the Veterans Affairs health system and managed care, have economic incentives that are better aligned for HaH adoption. Currently, HaH has been adopted by several Veterans Affairs health system and managed care systems. Development of a payment mechanism for HaH using a Medicare demonstration waiver is pending approval; if accomplished, this would spur HaH development, as it would require HaH model definition, quality and care standards, and model fidelity.[56]

HIGH-TECH HOME CARE

The term "high-tech home care" is used to describe a bevy of services, such as intravenous infusion therapy of antibiotics, total parenteral nutrition, chemotherapy, or analgesia. Additional "high-tech" services include home ventilators, oxygen therapy, home-based imaging, and telemedicine monitoring of chronic disease. These services are most commonly discussed in the context of home care services, or disease, care, and case management. When used on a long-term basis in the absence of acute illness, these do not constitute HaH care. However, these services and devices are often deployed by an HaH to treat acute illness in lieu of an acute hospital admission. As such technology continues to improve, it will permit the scope of HaH to expand and, in some cases, may reduce the need for on-site monitoring by medical personnel. For example, HaH staff could evaluate the need to visit an HaH patient with a complaint in the middle of the night by first observing the patient and listening to the heart and lungs via real-time video telemonitoring. During chronic care, these technological advances can improve access, quality, and coordination of care for medically complex community-dwelling older adults. We briefly review some of these technologies.

Recent advances in home intravenous infusion technologies allow infusion to be delivered in a highly controlled manner with programmable pumps,[57] also known as "smart pumps," with dose-checking capability, predefined dose limits, bolus delivery options, and the ability to recognize programming errors before medication delivery.[58] Pumps have evolved from large stationary units to portable devices that can be carried on a belt clip.[59] Ventilator technology has also moved from the inpatient setting to the home for patients with long-term ventilator requirements for a variety of disease processes,[60,61] including spinal cord injury and chronic lung disease. Descriptive studies suggest that home ventilation is a viable option with the expectation of successful weaning and survival with good quality-of-life outcomes.[62] In addition, these devices have become increasingly portable with some being the size of laptop computers, weighing as little as 13 lb.[63] Oxygen therapy has evolved[64] from reliance on bulky cylinders to safer, more compact, lightweight oxygen concentrators. Most concentrators can be plugged into a car's AC adaptor; others are battery powered and safe for outings or airplane travel. Simple home-based x-rays are available in many communities. Recently, handheld ultrasound devices have been developed, and they increase the feasibility of obtaining studies such as echocardiograms and diagnosing venous thrombosis or pleural, peritoneal, or pericardial fluid in the home-based patient.[65,66]

Telemedicine is a small but growing field with particular relevance to rural or homebound populations with chronic diseases that cannot otherwise access specialized care. Several types of specialty care, such as dermatology, ophthalmology, wound care, and treatment of infections,[67] have been studied in small clinical trials[68] and appear to allow accurate diagnosis and management through both real-time interactions and "store-and-forward" applications,[69] in which clinical data, including video images, are collected and stored for later review by a clinician. Similarly, home-based telemedicine interventions in chronic diseases probably enhance communication between patients and providers and facilitate closer monitoring of overall health when conducted in settings with specialized equipment and dedicated staff.[70,71] A recent systematic review of 65 studies of home telemonitoring for 4 chronic diseases (pulmonary conditions, diabetes, hypertension, and cardiovascular diseases) suggests that while telemonitoring is a promising patient-management approach, further studies are needed to examine its clinical effects and cost effectiveness.[72]

Although the evidence is limited by methodological variability, lack of comparison with in-person evaluation, and absence of clinical outcome measures, a recent systematic review by the Agency for Healthcare Research and Quality concluded that, in some situations, the use of telemedicine might be warranted even if the evidence is inconclusive, including "remote rural areas or other locations where medical care is not available locally and the patient is, for whatever reason, unable to travel to a setting where it can be obtained."[73] Additional small or methodologically weak trials are unlikely to greatly improve the evidence base, and larger, well-designed trials that include clinically meaningful outcomes are needed in light of increasing advocacy for payers to cover its use.

SUMMARY

Although the acute hospital is the standard venue for treating acute serious illness, it is often a difficult environment for older adults who are highly susceptible to functional decline and other iatrogenic consequences of hospital care. Hospital care is also expensive. Providing acute hospital-level care at home, in lieu of usual institutional care, is viable. As an emerging service model, the definition of HaH remains unsettled. Data favor HaH models that provide substantial physician inputs and are geared toward substituting for hospital care, provide service that is highly satisfying to patients and their caregivers, are associated with less iatrogenic complications, and are less expensive. Dissemination of HaH in integrated delivery systems is feasible. Widespread dissemination of HaH in the United States will require payment reform that acknowledges the role of HaH in the health care system.

ACKNOWLEDGMENT

The authors wish to thank Ms. Deborah Statom for assistance with manuscript preparation.

REFERENCES

1. Paulson HM Jr, Chao EL, et al. 2008 Annual report of the Boards of Trustees of the Federal hospital insurance and Federal supplementary medical insurance trust funds. Available at: http://www.cms.hhs.gov/reportstrustfunds/downloads/tr2008.pdf. 2008; [accessed September 16, 2008].
2. Kohn LT, Corrigan JM, Donaldson MS. To err is human: building a safer health system. Washington, DC: National Academy Press; 2000.
3. Leape LL, Berwick DM. Five years after to err is human: what have we learned? JAMA 2005;293(19):2384–90.
4. Leape LL, Brennan TA, Laird N, et al. The nature of adverse events in hospitalized patients. Results of the Harvard Medical Practice Study II. N Engl J Med 1991; 324(6):377–84.
5. Thomas EJ, Brennan TA. Incidence and types of preventable adverse events in elderly patients: population based review of medical records. BMJ 2000; 320(7237):741–4.
6. Brennan TA, Leape LL, Laird NM, et al. Incidence of adverse events and negligence in hospitalized patients. Results of the Harvard Medical Practice Study I. N Engl J Med 1991;324(6):370–6.
7. Creditor MC. Hazards of hospitalization of the elderly. Ann Intern Med 1993; 118(3):219–23.
8. Inouye SK, Bogardus ST Jr, Charpentier PA, et al. A multicomponent intervention to prevent delirium in hospitalized older patients. N Engl J Med 1999;340(9): 669–76.

9. Covinsky KE, Palmer RM, Fortinsky RH, et al. Loss of independence in activities of daily living in older adults hospitalized with medical illnesses: increased vulnerability with age. J Am Geriatr Soc 2003;51(4):451–8.

10. Coleman EA, Berenson RA. Lost in transition: challenges and opportunities for improving the quality of transitional care. Ann Intern Med 2004;141(7):533–6.

11. Forster AJ, Murff HJ, Peterson JF, et al. Adverse drug events occurring following hospital discharge. J Gen Intern Med 2005;20(4):317–23.

12. CMS feels the heat as consumers fume about Part D benefit services. Med Health 2006;60(26):1–2.

13. Quality Reports. CMS and JCAHO strive to help consumers make better healthcare decisions. Health Care Food Nutr Focus 2003;20(8):9.

14. Poretz DM. The infusion center: a model for outpatient parenteral antibiotic therapy. Rev Infect Dis 1991;13(Suppl 2):S142–6.

15. Grizzard MB, Harris G, Karns H. Use of outpatient parenteral antibiotic therapy in a health maintenance organization. Rev Infect Dis 1991;13(Suppl 2):S174–9.

16. Tice AD. An office model of outpatient parenteral antibiotic therapy. Rev Infect Dis 1991;13(Suppl 2):S184–8.

17. Tice AD, Marsh PK, Craven PC, et al. Home intravenous antibiotic therapy. Am J Med 1993;94(1):114–5.

18. Wolter JM, Bowler SD, Nolan PJ, et al. Home intravenous therapy in cystic fibrosis: a prospective randomized trial examining clinical, quality of life and cost aspects. Eur Respir J 1997;10(4):896–900.

19. Talcott JA, Whalen A, Clark J, et al. Home antibiotic therapy for low-risk cancer patients with fever and neutropenia: a pilot study of 30 patients based on a validated prediction rule. J Clin Oncol 1994;12(1):107–14.

20. Richards SH, Coast J, Gunnell DJ, et al. Randomised controlled trial comparing effectiveness and acceptability of an early discharge, hospital at home scheme with acute hospital care. BMJ 1998;316(7147):1796–801.

21. Shepperd S, Harwood D, Jenkinson C, et al. Randomised controlled trial comparing hospital at home care with inpatient hospital care. I: three month follow up of health outcomes. BMJ 1998;316(7147):1786–91.

22. Knowelden J, Westlake L, Wright KG, et al. Peterborough hospital at home: an evaluation. J Public Health Med 1991;13(3):182–8.

23. O'Cathain A. Evaluation of a hospital at home scheme for the early discharge of patients with fractured neck of femur. J Public Health Med 1994;16(2):205–10.

24. Rudd AG, Wolfe CD, Tilling K, et al. Randomised controlled trial to evaluate early discharge scheme for patients with stroke. BMJ 1997;315(7115):1039–44.

25. Rodgers H, Soutter J, Kaiser W, et al. Early supported hospital discharge following acute stroke: pilot study results. Clin Rehabil 1997;11(4):280–7.

26. Martin F, Oyewole A, Moloney A. A randomized controlled trial of a high support hospital discharge team for elderly people. Age Ageing 1994;23(3):228–34.

27. Cotton MM, Bucknall CE, Dagg KD, et al. Early discharge for patients with exacerbations of chronic obstructive pulmonary disease: a randomized controlled trial. Thorax 2000;55(11):902–6.

28. Davies L, Wilkinson M, Bonner S, et al. "Hospital at home" versus hospital care in patients with exacerbations of chronic obstructive pulmonary disease: prospective randomized controlled trial. BMJ 2000;321(7271):1265–8.

29. Skwarska E, Cohen G, Skwarski KM, et al. Randomized controlled trial of supported discharge in patients with exacerbations of chronic obstructive pulmonary disease. Thorax 2000;55(11):907–12.

30. Caplan GA, Ward JA, Brennan NJ, et al. Hospital in the home: a randomised controlled trial. Med J Aust 1999;170(4):156–60.
31. Aimonino Ricauda N, Tibaldi V, Leff B, et al. Substitutive "hospital at home" versus inpatient care for elderly patients with exacerbations of chronic obstructive pulmonary disease: a prospective randomized, controlled trial. J Am Geriatr Soc 2008;56(3):493–500.
32. Ricauda NA, Tibaldi V, Marinello R, et al. Acute ischemic stroke in elderly patients treated in hospital at home: a cost minimization analysis. J Am Geriatr Soc 2005; 53(8):1442–3.
33. Tibaldi V, Aimonino N, Ponzetto M, et al. A randomized controlled trial of a home hospital intervention for frail elderly demented patients: behavioral disturbances and caregiver's stress. Arch Gerontol Geriatr Suppl 2004;38(9):431–6.
34. Ricauda NA, Bo M, Molaschi M, et al. Home hospitalization service for acute uncomplicated first ischemic stroke in elderly patients: a randomized trial. J Am Geriatr Soc 2004;52(2):278–83.
35. Leff B, Burton L, Mader SL, et al. Comparison of stress experienced by family members of patients treated in hospital at home with that of those receiving traditional acute hospital care. J Am Geriatr Soc 2008;56(1):117–23.
36. Leff B, Burton L, Mader S, et al. Satisfaction with hospital at home care. J Am Geriatr Soc 2006;54(9):1355–63.
37. Leff B, Burton L, Mader SL, et al. Hospital at home: feasibility and outcomes of a program to provide hospital-level care at home for acutely ill older patients. Ann Intern Med 2005;143(11):798–808.
38. Wilson A, Parker H, Wynn A, et al. Randomised controlled trial of effectiveness of Leicester hospital at home scheme compared with hospital care. BMJ 1999; 319(7224):1542–6.
39. Jones J, Wilson A, Parker H, et al. Economic evaluation of hospital at home versus hospital care: cost minimisation analysis of data from randomised controlled trial. BMJ 1999;319(7224):1547–50.
40. Caplan GA, Coconis J, Woods J. Effect of hospital in the home treatment on physical and cognitive function: a randomized controlled trial. J Gerontol A Biol Sci Med Sci 2005;60(8):1035–8.
41. Board N, Brennan N, Caplan GA. A randomised controlled trial of the costs of hospital as compared with hospital in the home for acute medical patients. Aust N Z J Public Health 2000;24(3):305–11.
42. Leff B, Montalto M. Home hospital-toward a tighter definition. J Am Geriatr Soc 2004;52(12):2141.
43. Leff B. Acute care at home. The health and cost effects of substituting home care for inpatient acute care: a review of the evidence. J Am Geriatr Soc 2001;49(8):1123–5.
44. Shepperd S, Iliffe S. Hospital at home versus in-patient hospital care. Cochrane Database Syst Rev 2005;(3):CD000356.
45. Leff B, Burton L, Bynum JW, et al. Prospective evaluation of clinical criteria to select older persons with acute medical illness for care in a hypothetical home hospital. J Am Geriatr Soc 1997;45(9):1066–73.
46. Committee on the Future Health Care Workforce for Older Americans, Institute of Medicine. Retooling for an aging America: building the health care workforce. Report Brief 2008.
47. Melin AL, Bygren LO. Efficacy of the rehabilitation of elderly primary health care patients after short-stay hospital treatment. Med Care 1992;30(11):1004–15.
48. Coast J, Richards SH, Peters TJ, et al. Hospital at home or acute hospital care? A cost minimisation analysis. BMJ 1998;316(7147):1802–6.

49. Stessman J, Ginsberg G, Hammerman-Rozenberg R, et al. Decreased hospital utilization by older adults attributable to a home hospitalization program. J Am Geriatr Soc 1996;44(5):591–8.

50. Wilson A, Wynn A, Parker H. Patient and carer satisfaction with 'hospital at home': quantitative and qualitative results from a randomised controlled trial. Br J Gen Pract 2002;52(474):9–13.

51. Leff B, Burton L, Guido S, et al. Home hospital program: a pilot study. J Am Geriatr Soc 1999;47(6):697–702.

52. Leff B, Burton L, Mader S, et al. Functional outcomes associated with hospital at home care compared with traditional acute hospital care. J Am Geriatr Soc, in press.

53. Frick K, Burton L, Clark R, et al. Costs of hospital at home care versus traditional acute hospital care for older persons. Am J Manage Care, in press.

54. Rogers EM. Diffusion of Innovations. Washington, DC: The Free Press; 2003.

55. Campbell M, Fitzpatrick R, Haines A, et al. Framework for design and evaluation of complex interventions to improve health. BMJ 2000;321(7262):694–6.

56. Leff B. Dissemination of models of geriatric care: facilitators and barriers. 2007. Available at: http://www.iom.edu/Object.File/Master/43/860/Bruce%20Leff%20IOM%20Presentation%20SF%2006-28-07%20update.pdf. Accessed November 21, 2008.

57. Williams DN, Gibson JA, Bosch D. Home intravenous antibiotic therapy using a programmable infusion pump. Arch Intern Med 1989;149(5):1157–60.

58. Wilson K, Sullivan M. Preventing medication errors with smart infusion technology. Am J Health Syst Pharm 2004;61(2):177–83.

59. Delphi IVantage™ volumetric ambulatory infusion system. Available at: http://delphimedical.com/pdf/IVantageSellSheet.pdf. Accessed October 4, 2008.

60. Lewarski JS, Gay PC. Current issues in home mechanical ventilation. Chest 2007;132(2):671–6.

61. Lloyd-Owen SJ, Donaldson GC, Ambrosino N, et al. Patterns of home mechanical ventilation use in Europe: results from the Eurovent survey. Eur Respir J 2005;25(6):1025–31.

62. Salahuddin N, Haider K, Husain SJ, et al. Outcome of home mechanical ventilation. J Coll Physicians Surg Pak 2005;15(7):387–90.

63. VentWorld. Available at: http://www.ventworld.com/. Accessed October 4, 2008.

64. Gallegos LC, Shigeoka JW. Novel oxygen-concentrator-based equipment: take a test drive first!. Respir Care 2006;51(1):25–8.

65. Lapostolle F, Petrovic T, Lenoir G, et al. Usefulness of hand-held ultrasound devices in out-of-hospital diagnosis performed by emergency physicians. Am J Emerg Med 2006;24(2):237–42.

66. Galasko GI, Lahiri A, Senior R. Portable echocardiography: an innovative tool in screening for cardiac abnormalities in the community. Eur J Echocardiogr 2003;4(2):119–27.

67. Eron LJ, Marineau M, Baclig E, et al. The virtual hospital: treating acute infections in the home by telemedicine. Hawaii Med J 2004;63(10):291–3.

68. Johnston B, Wheeler L, Deuser J, et al. Outcomes of the Kaiser permanente tele-home health research project. Arch Fam Med 2000;9(1):40–5.

69. Moreno-Ramirez D, Ferrandiz L, Nieto-Garcia A, et al. Store-and-forward teledermatology in skin cancer triage: experience and evaluation of 2009 teleconsultations. Arch Dermatol 2007;143(4):479–84.

70. Artinian NT, Flack JM, Nordstrom CK, et al. Effects of nurse-managed telemonitoring on blood pressure at 12-month follow-up among urban African Americans. Nurse Res 2007;56(5):312–22.

71. Green BB, Cook AJ, Ralston JD, et al. Effectiveness of home blood pressure monitoring, web communication, and pharmacist care on hypertension control: a randomized controlled trial. J Am Med Assoc 2008;299(24):2857–67.

72. Pare G, Jaana M, Sicotte C. Systematic review of home telemonitoring for chronic diseases: the evidence base. J Am Med Inform Assoc 2007;14(3):269–77.

73. Telemedicine for the Medicare population—update. Available at: http://www.ahrq. gov/clinic/tp/telemeduptp.htm. Accessed September 14, 2008.

New Diagnostic and Information Technology for Mobile Medical Care

C. Gresham Bayne, MD, FAAEM[a],*, Peter A. Boling, MD[b]

KEYWORDS

- Point-of-care testing • House call technology
- Mobile medicine • Mobile clinician • Mobile physician
- House call technology • Electronic health records
- Health information technology

When my house is on fire, I don't ask 911 to send a doctor.
Why then, when my chest hurts, do I have to call the fireman?

An explosion of interest in mobile medical care is underway. Even before the Advanced Medical Home was described, physicians began making house calls using portable technologies for diagnosis, providing advanced procedures, and electronically documenting it all.

Before presenting these technologies, their clinical relevance, and their economic potentials, it is important to discuss the role of technology in mobile medical care. After 300,000 house calls in 6 states, our multispecialty group practice has learned that the elegant, but seemingly simple, concept of bringing care to the patient, rather than bringing the patient to the provider, involves numerous complex decisions and launches debates without precedent.

House calls are transformative, returning medicine to its origins when Hippocrates said, "and into whosoever's house I may enter, may I see the man—just the man." That should give us pause. Our practice calls it "the doorbell effect." Coming to the patient's home, especially with devices and skills that can avert a trip to the emergency room (ER), physicians cast themselves in a powerful light of trust and service. Patients are different: less wary, more comfortable. Yet there is danger. The dramatically restored doctor-patient relationship can lead to clinical shortcuts, accepted by both doctor and patient. We sometimes wait too long or do too little.

[a] Janus Health, 5030 Camino de la Siesta, Suite 405, San Diego, CA 92108, USA
[b] Virginia Commonwealth University, Richmond, VA, USA
* Corresponding author.
E-mail address: gbayne@janushealth.com (C.G. Bayne).

Clin Geriatr Med 25 (2009) 93–107
doi:10.1016/j.cger.2008.10.007
0749-0690/08/$ – see front matter © 2009 Published by Elsevier Inc.

geriatric.theclinics.com

Imagine confronting the difficulty of arranging an imaging study in a spastic, quadriplegic, cerebral palsy patient with poorly described neck pain weeks after a fall from his wheelchair. Great effort was required to convince this patient that he needed a neck computed tomographic (CT) scan, which showed an unstable fracture requiring 2-level fusion. The cautionary tale reminds us that patients who depend on house calls have such longstanding, heavy disease burden that they become "therapeutically nihilistic" and can make us co-dependent. Whether a diagnostic test is done, or not, should always be based on clinical need; one should not yield to complacency, nor should possessing a profitable technology encourage its use. This is just as true in house calls as in the clinic.

The authors' group practice has used portable technology for diagnostic testing in the home for nearly 30 years. Yet the evaluation of the impact and cost-benefit of these technologies remains empiric. There is a lack of refereed studies on outcomes from use of portable medical devices at home. Fortunately, the idea of high-tech physician house calls has attracted venture capital and allowed the authors' practice to explore new modalities. Some of them have been found to be overly costly or cumbersome.

There were surprises. Consider the blood count. For 10 years, a device such as a Coulter counter was used to perform complete blood counts during house calls. The hemoglobin value was often essential and may have saved lives. However, the white blood count had no impact on the care plan after the visit. Patients with surgical abdomens were hospitalized whether the white count was elevated, shifted, or not. Patients who were stable but had an elevated white count were treated the same as if the white count was unknown due to an abundance of caution taken with these frail elderly patients.

It was learned during the first decade of the authors' practice (the 1980s) that the only valuable point-of-care tests were those that affected disposition at the time of the home visit rather than diagnosis. House call physicians rely on the original skills in medicine, which makes them excellent clinicians: taking a careful history, performing an accurate exam, and then taking a good history again. Yet the new, inexpensive, portable testing devices expand the range of home care to include urgent care and even emergencies when they are needed.

There is much to be gained from this advanced care model. Reducing ER overcrowding is one potential benefit from urgent house calls. ERs are overwhelmed, with 110,000,000 visits expected this year. For most patients whose emergencies are not critical, the "golden hour" is now spent in the waiting room. This issue is more prevalent in low-income urban areas: for every $10,000 reduction in mean income for a community, there is a 10-minute increase in ER waiting time.[1]

The use of portable diagnostics is inherent to cost-effective care when patients are complex and illness is acute, and this should apply to the concentration of Medicare spending in a small percentage of beneficiaries: the 10% that consume nearly two-thirds of the Medicare budget. These patients have extensive comorbidity and multiple providers without centralized communication or timely access, thus leading to frequent trips to the hospital. Although patients receive thorough emergent care for acute episodes, care would be better and less costly if the cycle of disconnected urgent encounters in high-cost environments were disrupted. Even without portable diagnostics, Grade B evidence supports cost-effectiveness of the "hospital at home" model, taking patients diagnosed in the ER who qualified for inpatient care and providing both nursing and physician visits in the home.[2]

The emergency medicine literature is replete with descriptive studies showing that less than 20% of ER patients need immediate physician attention. The question is which ones are they? We know that the elderly are more likely to be admitted to the hospital once they arrive in the ER than younger patients, that patients arriving by ambulance are more likely to be admitted, and that the elderly take ambulances more often. Many states such as California have laws that require 911 to direct patients to the "nearest appropriate facility," which may be a medical center where the patient has no records and their doctor has no privileges.

According to Outcome and Assessment Information Set (OASIS)-B home health care data, more than 25% of Medicare home health patients use emergency care, yet in a convenience sample of one, a physician in the authors' house call group referred 104 consecutive new patients to a single home health agency in San Diego, and only three patients went to the ER during the home health benefit (one went twice).

From the perspective of a patient with an urgent medical need, the standard of care today is heavily influenced by factors that direct them to the hospital ER, where they do not want to go as their doctor often has no privileges and their medical records are seldom available to prevent unnecessary testing or procedures. A strong case for change can be built on the premise that the ER is an expensive site for primary care, while growing saturation problems threaten the very stability of regional emergency medical services (EMS) care for true emergencies.

Suppose that the basic diagnostic tests usually done in the ER were done during house calls, with a proper triage and dispatch system to protect emergently ill patients from delays. In the classic scenario, "I've fallen and I can't get up," a few questions asked over the phone tell us that hip pain, not chest pain, is the central issue. In fact, the American 911 system is based on "Clausen Cards" (after Jeff Clausen, EMS Director of Seattle Heart Watch). One of roughly three dozen chief complaints is selected, four or fewer yes/no questions are asked, and a dispatcher can correctly place the patient in the non-life-threatening category.

If the house call clinician can obtain timely portable x-rays and a few dispositive laboratory tests, it might be reasonable to see this patient at home, even on the floor, and do an x-ray to evaluate the hip. Imagine: the nonfractured patient is treated at home, and the fractured patient can be directly admitted after relevant medical conditions are also evaluated on the spot. Beginning in 1985, the authors' practice began seeing bedbound patients with osteoporotic hip fractures. Now, their hip fracture films are electronically sent to an orthopedist who sometimes elects to let nonambulatory patients with limited pain heal at home, avoiding the risks of fat embolism, delirium, and iatrogenic infections.

This scenario may raise questions. Office-based physicians will not know how happy this care makes patients and caregivers. ER physicians might argue that patients are inappropriately denied adequate care. The health maintenance organization gatekeeper may question the x-ray that costs $236 (Medicare charges). However, if you ask patients, most prefer to avoid the hospital or surgical suite if possible, and virtually all prefer direct admission to the ward, bypassing the ER.

SPECIFIC POINT-OF-CARE DIAGNOSTICS
Imaging

Although there is no consensus, community standard, or even parameters for proper debate about the concept of having control over the ordering and timely return of portable x-rays, a priori, the practice itself has a strong clinical rationale that is familiar to most facility-based clinicians who routinely order such x-rays every day.

Fortunately, Medicare payment makes x-ray the one profitable point-of-care ancillary, tied to a single code (R0070, transportation of x-ray), which is a "C" or carrier-rated code. In most areas of the country, this code is reimbursed at more than

$100, which makes physician-owned portable x-ray fiscally feasible. Entrepreneurs take note: a carrier-rated code may be changed at any time, and no national Medicare coverage policy exists as of late 2008. The capital expense of a portable x-ray service is also significant, and most states require the physician to have a Radiation Supervisor's Certificate, unless one employs certified radiology technologists.

Point-of-care testing with diagnostic x-rays improves timely care, but full value is realized only when the images can be electronically captured and transmitted in the mobile environment. Having spent two decades hiring couriers to drive films all over the two counties for "wet-reads," the authors urge all to consider this carefully. They now pay a monthly lease fee for a digital x-ray processor, couriers are no longer needed, and positive cash flow exists. Success hinges on volume and health information technology (HIT), discussed below.

Risk tolerance is a factor in deciding whether to invest in mobile x-ray technology. Medicare is looking ever more closely at costly technologies, starting with utilization of CT, magnetic resonance imaging (MRI), and positron emission tomographic and single photon emission computed tomographic scans. The worsening Medicare funding crisis may accelerate restrictions. Moreover, it is difficult to argue an established community standard, because there is no defined norm for the percentage of house calls that should involve a portable x-ray. In the authors' practice, 8% to 10% is typical, as much urgent care is provided. The frequency depends on providers' skills along with comfort reading films if they cannot find a radiologist to read them for the small Medicare professional fee (under $9).

A mention should be made of the portable MRI scanner (www.magnevu.com). This is a portable 500-gauss magnetometer, which could be brought into a patient's home and used in extremity exams. It is not yet in practical use due to issues such as the risk of pulling a metal file cabinet down on top of someone's grandchild and high capital cost.

Portable ultrasound machines such as the SonoSite (www.sonosite.com) or Cypress (http://www.imaging.com/acuson-cypress.html) are routinely used by emergency physicians for quick-look diagnosis of conditions such as gallstones or hemoperitoneum. For at least a decade, some house call physicians have also used ultrasound. Medicare policy on payment for ultrasound at home is rapidly changing, and rigid requirements can be anticipated for formal credentialing in reading or performing such studies. Ultrasound image quality depends on the technologist, and hospitals now pay ultrasonographers handsomely, so this point-of-care instrument could become unaffordable for the home-based practice, where the daily service volume is low. This is unfortunate, because the reliability of newer, high-resolution machines makes them easier to use and more powerful as a dispositive tool. Regardless of this, constraints on Medicare reimbursement should prompt a practice to do a thorough business analysis before investing in mobile ultrasound, and those who have invested must take care not to overutilize the devices to defray capital costs.

Beside the need for imaging, a common reason for physicians to send acutely ill homebound patients to the ER is need for timely laboratory work. Yet only a few laboratory tests have dispositive value, helping to decide if the patient needs facility-based care. This triage decision also depends on the confidence and skills of the practitioner, presence or absence of reliable emergency transport, ability of care systems to treat acute conditions in the home, and a reliable on-call physician when things do not go as expected.

As described earlier, the white blood cell count is useful but usually not critical for decision making. However, hemoglobin level, coagulation parameters (prothrombin time/international normalized ratio [PT/INR]), and blood gas testing may separate sick patients into one group that can receive outpatient care in the home and another group that requires hospitalization. Without laboratory tests, a report of melena usually results in an ER visit. Sometimes, confirming the low hemoglobin produces the same result. However, consider a pale anemic patient who has melena and a hemoglobin test result of 6 g/dL on point-of-care testing, but who is hemodynamically stable, old, and frail, with a signed do-not-resuscitate order and short life expectancy, and is at high risk for in-hospital complications. If the mobile clinician could use a nasogastric tube in the home to check for an upper GI bleed and had reliable home health agency support for telemedicine, transfusion, and twice daily laboratory monitoring, as in the authors' practice, might the decision-making change?

Suppose that a blood gas test is done at home to assess oxygenation in a lung cancer patient with pneumonia and it showed severe respiratory failure with a pH of 7.14, while the patient or family declined hospital care. Would the prognostic information help in counseling the family regarding imminent death and palliative care strategies? Conversely, might a similar patient with hypoxia, but no acidosis, be managed comfortably at home with oxygen and antibiotics?

Oximetry at home using fingertip pulse oximeters (www.nonin.com) has become widespread and provides one of the most useful bits of data for home care clinicians. Conversely, ongoing transcutaneous monitoring of oxygen or CO_2 is not seeing much use in home care due to cost, complexity, and limited availability of instrumentation and sensors, though this too could change. Overnight diagnostic oximetry (store-and-forward) is widely used as a screening test for oxygen therapy. As of this writing, a National Carrier Decision by the Centers for Medicare and Medicaid Services has authorized payment for home sleep apnea studies enabling continuous positive airway pressure therapies without requiring an overnight study at a sleep center.

Blood chemistry testing can be done with a single cartridge designed for the iSTAT machine (www.abbott.com). The iSTAT, which is licensed by the Clinical Laboratory Improvement Amendments (CLIA) program, has been used in house call practices for more than a decade. The moderately complex iSTAT device using an EC-8 cartridge provides the following values in 2 minutes: Na, K, Cl, HCO_3, BUN, Glu, Hgb, pH, and PCO_2 with calculated hematocrit, base excess, and anion gap. Additional cartridges are available for PT/INR, troponin I, beta naturetic peptide, myoglobin, and creatinine. Cartridges cost from $2 to $12 except for the cardiac tests, which cost about $40. Recent CLIA rules now include the iSTAT CHEM8 cartridge (similar to the EC-8 but with calcium and without the blood gases), for use under a CLIA waiver, lowering costs for the moderately complex testing status required up until November 2007.

One other potentially viable field chemistry analyzer is the Biosite Cardioprofiler, but to the authors' knowledge, no one has adopted it in the home setting. This machine (www.biosite.com) measures the main cardiac isoenzymes and myoglobin but is bigger, is less portable, and costs more per test than the iSTAT.

Cardiac bioimpedance is another test that has entered the mobile medical practice environment. The leading cause of death is heart disease, and home care clinicians manage congestive heart failure in a large number of patients, many of whom cannot give an accurate history. Thus, physiologic testing is valuable for fluid and medication management. The test measures total thoracic fluid using electrophysical properties. Although it is currently not often used, modern studies that find cardiac output measured by impedance comparable to thermodilution catheter data support using the test for ER and ICU settings, and point-of-care use in house calls has been described.[3]

The latest "black bag" can streamline the advanced house call by acquiring digital blood pressure, pulse, spirometry, oximetry, and imaging data through the same unified software package and integrate it with the chart (www.QRSdiagnostics.com, **Fig. 1**). Development of this care model is slowed by capital cost and inadequate

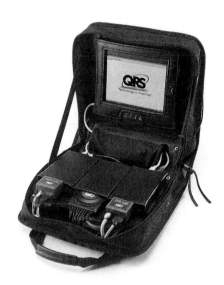

Fig. 1. Mobile Diagnostic Kit.

reimbursement under Medicare fee-for-service. Medicare reimbursement for point-of-care laboratory testing is the same as for tests run in a large-facility laboratory and drawn by the home health nurse; this fact and the high unit cost of portable tests ensure that providers doing point-of-care tests are doing it for purely clinical reasons and not for profit.

Most blood testing in home care is less urgent and can be done with samples correctly obtained, stored, and transported to a central location. The $3 venipuncture reimbursement from Medicare falls far short of costs incurred in obtaining and transporting blood samples, but this remains the most common approach in home medical care. Here, consider the cost of a physician obtaining and transporting a blood sample: $15 or more, conservatively assuming that this service adds 10 minutes, and the base physician cost is $100 per hour. This comparison makes the cost of point-of-care testing seem modest. Gain-sharing incentives under alternative payment models may correct this. For now, point-of-care testing works for the authors' practice, but a complete financial model with amortization of capital and maintenance costs for a moderately complex physician-owned laboratory under CLIA should be done before undertaking portable laboratory testing.

THE IMPORTANCE OF HIT COMMUNICATIONS

Today, there are several basic electronic medical record (EMR) systems in which home care providers record, report, and remotely access text documents and database information. Many home health agencies use this approach, and some medical practices are using EHR systems that were designed for office practices and are thus far from optimal but can capture the main elements of the encounter. However, the available systems are limited, and those limitations will soon be much more evident.

Understanding and using HIT is vital to the mobile clinician. The federal government is moving to increase reimbursement for those using HIT and has exempted physicians from Stark constraints on receiving support for HIT from a collaborative Designated Health Service (DHS).[4]

As of October 2008, the Energy and Commerce Subcommittee on Health is editing the "PROTECT 2009" Health Information Technology bill, and HIT is cited as a key strategy for purchasing better care and ultimately saving money in many health care reform proposals. On June 3, 2008, the U.S. Department of Health and Human Services published the Federal Health IT Strategic Plan 2008-2012.[5] Due to the input from the American Academy of Home Care Physicians, one of 25 strategic initiatives (Strategy 1.3.9) reads

"Remove technical, financial, workflow, and other barriers to diagnosing, treating, and communicating with patients outside the boundaries of traditional health care settings."

As part of the controversial Physician Fee Fix law passed and signed in July 2008 (H.R. 6331), e-prescribing physician quality measures were separated from the Physician Quality Reporting Initiatives (PQRI) program, and net bonuses of up to 2% within the next 4 years were authorized for physicians doing a majority of their prescribing by electronic means.[6,7] If a physician has not provided for e-prescribing by 2012, he or she will face a pay cut that scales up to 2%. This 4% spread applies to all Medicare payments to the physician; obviously, the federal government is serious about HIT.

HIT development is expensive. Some describe it as a $260 billion mandate on the medical professions, which has slowed its adoption rates and forced physicians in small practices to have corporate partners (eg, hospitals). Moreover, home health agencies and physicians have historically been limited in data sharing by prohibitions under earlier versions of anti-kickback and Stark rules. The pressing need for HIT led to another recent Final Rule, which allows a third party, even one receiving referrals from physicians, to pay 85% of physicians' HIT cost, including network administration, software, and communication technologies. Below this new Stark Exemption for HIT is summarized.

EHR EXCEPTION TO THE STARK RULES

The 2006 publication of the e-prescribing and health record Safe Harbors was associated with publication in FR 71 (152) on August 8, 2006 of the Final Rule for the exception to prohibitions on self-referrals inherent in both Stark rules and the anti-kickback statute. The definition of **"electronic health record"** is now federalized as

"A repository of consumer health status information in computer processable form used for clinical diagnosis and treatment for a broad array of clinical conditions."

The definition of **"interoperability"** is

"at the time of the donation, the software is able to (1) communicate and exchange data accurately, effectively, securely, and consistently with different information technology systems, software, applications, and networks, in various settings, and (2) exchange data such that the clinical or operational purpose and meaning of the data are preserved and unaltered."

For background, a Safe Harbor is a *voluntary* program, which requires submitting a request to the Office of Inspector General requesting formal written approval. The process requires revealing potential proprietary interests and "locks in" the program's attributes. Subsequent change in the relationship could put this Safe Harbor at risk. By contrast, seeking exception from self-referral rules is *mandatory*; failure to comply can result in felony penalties.

Section 3312 in the August 2006 Final Rule broadens Safe Harbor restrictions and unifies requirements for donating EMR and e-prescribing software under one rule. There is no support for hardware, but software and network supports are broadly defined. Key features are

1. A **Donor** can be any provider of DHSs as well as skilled nursing facilities (SNFs), assisted living facility, laboratories, pharmacies, radiation oncology centers, Alzheimer Day Centers, Health Plans, Regional Health Information Organizations (RHIOs), dialysis facilities, and other entities that "enhance the overall health of a community."
2. Any physician or member of a medical group, contractor or not, is an eligible **Recipient**, but not an SNF, ALF, laboratory, DME provider, pharmacy, Physician Hospital Organization, RHIO, health plan, clinical laboratory, network provider, or other entities that "operate, support, or manage network providers."
3. The technology company does not have to be a signatory to the donor/recipient contract; all "forms of connectivity services" are covered by the Exception but hardware is not.
4. The primary purpose of the donated HIT must be of clinical merit and constitute the majority of provided services, although general supportive functionality can be included (eg, a scheduling function that can schedule private or personal meetings along with patient encounters).
5. The donated services must include e-prescribing, and a separate e-Rx Exception was not created for this final Rule, unlike the 2 Safe Harbors.
6. "Prescription information" is defined as "information about prescriptions for drugs or any other item or service normally accomplished through a written prescription."
7. There is a requirement to comply "with the applicable standards under Medicare Part D at the time the items and services are donated."
8. There is no restriction on commercial messaging or formulary compliance, which are considered "free speech."
9. Routers or modems are not protected.
10. Data migration is not required to prior or future software services.
11. Although donated services may be "deemed" by having a Certification Committee for Health Information Technology (CCHIT) or other appropriate certification, they are not required to be so certified; however, they must be "interoperable, given the prevailing state of technology at the time the items or services are provided to the physician recipient." Parties should have a "reasonable basis for determining that software is interoperable" to avoid uncertainty.

The specific, listed requirements for the Exception are

1. Protects software, IT, and training used predominantly "to create, maintain, transmit, or receive EHRs"
2. Must be interoperable as defined in 411.351
3. Must contain e-prescribing functionality or interface with the physician's current e-prescribing solution
4. All categories of DHS may donate to any physician

5. Physician selection cannot take into consideration the volume or value of referrals
6. There is no limitation in value of the donated services, but the physician must pay 15% of the fair market value
7. Donor's cost must be documented in the agreement and precludes replacing similar physician services
8. Use of donated IT must be without regard to pay or status for any patient
9. Sunsets on New Year's Eve 2013 (thus requiring review of the policy)

TECHNICAL PROBLEMS UNIQUE TO THE MOBILE PROVIDER

There are 3 main areas of difficulty when attempting to build a fully operational mobile EHR. First is the Health Insurance Portability and Accountability Act (HIPAA) requirement for security of records and complexity of wireless connectivity. Second is compliance with Stark rules. Third is functionality in real-life practice. **Table 1** contains an important lexicon.

HIPAA Considerations

As one of the few doctors who read the entire HIPAA statute, the author (C.G.B) can verify that the word "reasonable" occurs 52 times. For example, one should take "reasonable" steps to protect privacy. A small medical group or solo practice has fewer barriers to compliance. If you operate in a virtual private network (VPN) with 128-bit encryption, you are probably HIPAA-compliant, as long as you meet other requirements, such as automatically turning off your computer after it is unattended for 15 minutes.

However, you cannot be HIPAA-compliant if you save data on your client computer without encrypting them. If someone finds your computer, even password-protected through VPN controls, they can take your hard drive, put it in another computer, and read patient records (plus your private folders).

Table 1 Common terms used in networks	
MB/s	Per second transmission speed in megabytes (8 million bits)/s
Kb/sec	Kilobyte per second transmission speed (8,000 bits/s)
Byte/bit	A Byte is equal to 8 bits (the "B" is typically capitalized in Byte)
Client	The mobile user's computer
Server	The office-based computer connecting to a client
Thin client	Client must be connected to the server's application to function
Fat client	Client where application resides both on server and client
VPN	A virtual private network meeting electronic privacy standards
Upload	The process of sending data from the client to the server
Download	The process of sending data from the server to the client
WLAN	A wireless local area (in-building) network meeting 802.11x standards
WiFi	A small area wireless network, usually confined to a building, allowing broadband speeds of 10–100 MB/s
WWAN	A true wireless network covering a wide area within a city or larger, allowing broadband speeds of .050-.800 MB/s to upload and slightly faster to download
DS3	A scalable network speed allowing variable expansion of broadband to meet demand
CCHIT	Certification Committee for Health Information Technology

Current Legislation

Congress is currently considering or enacting legislation for health care reform that hinges on HIT application, including expanded funds for the Advanced Medical Home demonstration, the Independence at Home Act introduced in October 2008, and bonus payments for PQRI and e-prescribing. It is likely that current voluntary compliance with a certification of your EMR or network will soon become compulsory (see www.cchit.org for the standards).

However, fully developed mobile charting or e-prescribing is incompatible with design characteristics built into the CCHIT process. Proposed CCHIT requirements are based on office and institutional settings, where a cabled desktop computer can interact with the database at 10 to 100 MB/s speeds. A mobile provider virtually never has that opportunity. Thus, although the Safe Harbors offer a funding mechanism for expanded home care HIT, the performance standards are inconsistent with system response time.

PQRI measures are easily built into an EMR or other computerized database for mobile medical care. However, PQRI was designed for office practice, and only 19 of the 138 original measures had the home visit and rest home CPT codes attached. In 2009, 15 more measures will be included, with the home visit codes for eligibility finally added after strong input from the American Academy of Home Care Physicians (AAHCP) and support from the American Medical Association (AMA).

EHR FUNCTIONALITY

Today's problems lie hidden just beneath the surface. Only a few EMRs can operate in a mobile environment, and these often cannot cope with asynchronicity (when the wireless signal is suddenly dropped while driving around). Most significantly, the plethora of e-prescribing handheld devices have created a special "always connected at broadband" standard, which mobile tablet computers cannot integrate due to the aforementioned slow bandwidth and special SCRIPT communication language unique to the e-prescribing industry.

Consider house call scenarios with multiple providers using the system at once. Assume that you have a standard EVDO, version A, G3 wireless modem in your laptop and a typical chart is 2 MB (common even without images). Your wireless carrier claims to support transmissions up to 10 MB/s, but this applies only to "bursts" during the downloading of files (think Napster or YouTube). The greatest need in mobile practices is uploading charts to the server. EVDO modems upload at much slower rates.

The authors' group uses a wireless modem with maximum upload capability advertised by the vendor as 10 Mb/s. However, when 8 clinicians are working and the office staff are receiving and sending messages, the network's VPN digital pipe (a robust DS3 capable of handling traffic from 30 T1 lines) can be of almost limitless capacity, but one must still wait for data to pass through the chokepoint of the wireless vendor's system. The vendors give about 0.115 MB/s upload speeds and 0.6-2.0 MB/s download speeds that depend on the number of other wireless users at that moment. Think of all 14-year-olds getting out of school at the same time and downloading high-intensity videogames and tunes. A 2-MB digital file can be sent in three minutes at typical speeds and received in 50 seconds. Both are too slow for efficient mobile medical care as one has to sit waiting to avoid sudden disconnects that result from driving. As a result, one must limit individual encounter files to several kilobytes, not 2 MB, for facile charting using a wireless modem.

This is particularly difficult with digital x-rays. Even with Digital Imaging and Communications in Medicine compression software in a PACS system, a chest x-ray has about 10 to 30 MB of data. With EVDO wireless modem upload speeds of 0.115

MB/s, sending a chest x-ray from a client to the server would take 45 minutes! EHR companies have not addressed this problem because fiberoptic systems in clinics send large x-ray files in three seconds (at 10-100 MB/s). Policymakers are just becoming acquainted with mobile networking problems, and the AAHCP is working to prevent new rulesthat would preclude mobile clinicians from ever meeting the standards.

Though chart upload transmission speed is one critical issue, there are others. File system auditing software allows you to find lost files and track when any file was accessed and by whom. This capability is required by both CCHIT and HIPAA and is needed by clinicians for obvious reasons. For example, during an audit or malpractice claim, it is critical that you can prove files were not altered after the fact. Currently, this software alone would cost over $3,000 per member if purchased for the mobile medical group.

Finally, if you have more than two providers on your EHR, you will need a network. This separates the boutique practice from those that have scaled in size. It requires not only a major capital investment in hardware and software but ongoing IT support or "network administration." This is the most expensive part of the future, although it could soon save money. In addition, do not forget: network administration costs a provider group about 20% of the capital cost of each EMR user every year.

Think of this like putting your medical practice on the information highway. If you buy a car (EHR), you want the best car for the least price and only those extras (horsepower, tires, and accessories) that you need for the kind of driving you do. Once on the road, you want to avoid driving on a bumpy dirt road (unstable network). Salespersons are promoting "road ready" EHRs but beware: if the EHR is complex, you may not be able to participate in a network that can accommodate the EMR or use its features. Remember, it is not the EHR but the network that is most difficult to maintain and is expensive!

WHAT IS THE SOLUTION?

The AAHCP is seeking to educate the CCHIT standards-writing consortium (www.cchit.org). The EHR industry is large and competitive, and digital records may soon be mandated, so vendors must address asynchronous (store-and-forward) issues and slow wireless transmission rates. For now, the solo physician or two-person team can function adequately with basic laptops and "save-as" features with standard small-size text documents, using Outlook for communications. To achieve some, but not all, important EHR features using existing wireless information architecture, a digital record can be made to meet the certification standards by the network you use.

Seek to make sure your network uses a packet such as XML, which allows transmission of your chart entries onto a chart template at the client and the server, rather than requiring transmission of the whole chart each time. One can think of having a Christmas tree in the office and another on the tablet: ornaments are hung on the tree by entering data on the tablet; the same tree exists in the office but only ornaments need to be uploaded.

Mobile Computers: the menu of computer options is beyond the scope of this article, but certain points should be made. Mobile diagnosticians must decide about screen pixel density and size for reviewing EKGs or images. The author believes reading an EKG or wet-reading a chest x-ray can be safely done only with an 8×11-inch screen, which pushes one into the high-end tablet market. Remember, you may find value in "wet-reading" an x-ray on an iPhone, but ultimately your malpractice insurer and payers will require the reading of films with adequate screen size, pixel density, and PACS safeguards.

Systems using e-mail, dictation, and charting software are evolving for blackberries and other handheld devices. These "constantly on" Internet devices use a separate wireless Internet stream and are easier to carry and use than a fully loaded tablet computer. Newer systems allow voice streaming over the Internet for transcription, but take caution: wave files require so much bandwidth that full HIPAA compliance measures are unlikely to be available for such high-end services.

HIPAA requires complex encryption protocols both on transmitted data and on the data received and/or stored on the portable device, so handheld devices suffer heat-dissipation barriers, making them literally too hot to handle, even when newer chips are able to process the required data loads. Generally, the heat problem is a more limiting factor in mobile medicine than is battery life, because one can plug into home or vehicle power sources between visits.

In sum, as of October 2008 none of over 300 CCHIT-certified EMRs offers on-line functionality in a house call practice due to the high-broadband, "constantly on" designs. CCHIT requires robust connections for applications such as automatic cross-checks for billing compliance, selecting ICD-9 codes, and real-time drug-utilization-review checks with cost comparison data for generics. These functions are beyond the scope of wireless hardware integrated with a usable mobile electronic record and communication system. The "store-and-forward" solutions touted by vendors are misleading because few physicians can remember to toggle on and off the Internet when they are near WiFi broadband connections that meet HIPAA standards.

Surprisingly, this leaves wireless communication as the most important discussion of new technologies for the mobile physician. Considering the foregoing, there are 3 available strategies to design HIT solutions:

1. Take notes and enter data at the end of the day or when connected to the Internet; this is now the most common approach.
2. Enter data on a fat client portable device, and synchronize data at points of the day when able to obtain a fast WiFi or cable connection; generally, this is done in academic centers or where a hospital has donated HIT to a mobile practice contracted with the institution. The author calls this the "Starbucks practice" after the first ubiquitous chain that had T-Mobile WiFi access in most stores…plus coffee.
3. Design around the slow wireless wide area network (WWAN) upload speeds and make concessions on data content to allow fully-automated, real-time functionality (Disclosure: the author is a principal in www.janushealth.com, which claims to be the only vendor for this service)

Ultimately, the critical issue for mobile clinical computing is not cost, which dominates most current publications, nor ease of use. It is wide-area-network broadband speed, with upload being more limiting than download, especially with diagnostic imaging. The 3G, EVDO, Version (A) modems in cell phones and portable tablet computers are all too slow for full functionality, whether with Sprint, Verizon, AT&T, or other wireless services.

Slow connection speed has clinical implications. In collaborations with home health agencies and others, whether for the Advanced Medical Home, Independence at Home, or other models, the ability to store and forward a physician note and an order for a hypothetical patient whose hemoglobin is 6 g/dL is not the only problem. The crux is when the order is uploaded to the Internet and downloaded by the home health nurse tasked with safeguarding the patient by transfusion, close monitoring, and follow-up testing. It is too risky to rely on provider memory to frequently "toggle on" to the Internet, and secure wireless options are still too slow. So for now, less efficient methods are used, sharing time-sensitive communications via pager, landlines, or cellular phones.

"Sassy" New Models: Big problems arise when you shift from solo mobile practice to group practice. Even with one associate, the scalable need for cross-coverage, chart sharing, and common working files leads quickly to requiring network administration and business associates who understand the cost, maintenance, and repair of Internet-enabled communication systems. Until recently, this was cost-prohibitive to most small medical groups. Now, designers offer software-as-a-service (SAAS), which helps avoid the capital cost of software and network creation (colocation, disaster recovery, and so on). Fee rates are calculated per encounter or per megabyte of data and become scalable with the revenue stream of a growing practice.

SAAS models may seem far afield in a treatise on home care but are ultimately critical to creating an appealing practice model and solving workforce problems. Analogy to an apartment house is helpful. The typical EMR represents a finished product such as a condominium building with huge development costs and resistance to change. Tenants pay a deposit (capital expense for software) and monthly rent (license fees) for the right to use the space and utilities controlled by the landlord. There are periodic infrastructure upgrades and often unsolicited condominium association fees to cover new features such as a HVAC heater or earthquake protection (source code updates for the EHR). Once built, infrastructure tends to remain in the apartment until it breaks, because replacement is expensive, and you have little control over getting new services specific to your apartment.

In a SAAS condominium, you could pay no up-front capital expense with one all-inclusive monthly fee, which covers all obvious and hidden costs, such as utilities, upgrades, new capital equipment, maintenance, and breakdowns. The fee is contracted, cannot change during the term, and may be priced innovatively, such as paying "for every time you walk into your apartment" or "for every hour you are in your apartment." If you want to paint your apartment purple (change the EMR macros), you pay the cost of doing it and do not need permission from other tenants, just the landlord. If you want to save money by renting a smaller room (ie, no x-ray capability), you can renegotiate fees in the middle of your contract, since all ongoing expenses are already capitalized, and the building is unlikely to burn down. If it did burn down, you have no loss, because you simply stop paying the fees for a service that can no longer be provided, although one might expect major reorganization costs by going back to paper or purchasing an alternative mobile EHR.

SAAS architecture will become the computing model for small groups of physicians, because few have the capital or desire to build an HIT network. A great advantage is that SAAS allows fully autonomous physicians to acquire HIT without having their charts and practices "captured" by a hospital donating HIT because physicians cannot afford it.

The broadband wireless modem speed problem will not be solved soon, but numerous products and services will continue proffering false claims of immediate cures. Exciting new portable devices will be seen, from a handheld device to replace mammography, to friendly human sensing devices (www.philometron.com), to the talking cane (which tells you how you are progressing with physical therapy after your total hip arthroplasty). Many will fail; others will transform markets. Today, what is needed to practice quality medicine in the home is available and replaces a trip to the ER for the vast majority of patients; all that is needed now is for someone to increase the speed of light so that the wireless modem will work better!

Telemedicine

Point-of-care testing has long been connected to home telemonitors, which can acquire data and stream them over a telephone line or modem. Typically, the parameters being tracked include pulse oximetry, vital signs, cardiac rhythm, and daily weights, when they can be reliably obtained in the home. These "boxes," or "PC Hubs" as IBM calls them, are designed to connect patients with electronic health information systems and stream data into various downstream revenue pools, pharmacies being the most prevalent.

Little has been done in design and development to account for the additional functional needs of a mobile clinician visiting patients at the time of their illness. The telemonitoring industry has been built to address remote (rural) signal transmission, such as teleradiology or live streaming of patient interviews. In remote settings where travel time to the home is a serious logistic issue, the high cost and broadband utilization required for a patient to view the interviewing physician may make sense. In other settings, one could argue that it is settling for second best when one can practically have in-person contact.

A current focus of telemedicine is arrhythmia management. Numerous methods exist for sending simple digital EKG rhythm strips over a telephone or modem to a monitoring call center, where a registered nurse or high-tech alarm system identifies suspect patterns, captures them in digital memory, and alerts the physician on his or her office computer or tablet. Of these, CardioNet (www.cardionet.com) is the most developed and used.

Home care patients suffer from multiple diseases, and dementia is prevalent. When choosing telemonitoring services, one must consider a service that can be used passively. Innovative passive systems, such as LifeShirt (www.LifeShirt.com), apply a garment with electrodes, worn by a bedbound patient, that acquire signals for cardiac impedance and pulse. As the price drops, these may see more use.

Get ready for sensing technologies using lasers, spectroscopy, impedance, monoclonal antibodies, and other noninvasive measures that are being developed for cancer detection, laboratory values without blood sampling, point-of-care microbiology, and remote monitoring through radiofrequency (RF) devices costing less than $8. In 1985, accurate cardiac outputs were measured in the University of California San Diego LifeFlight helicopter while transporting trauma patients, and Mayo Clinic Aerovac teams were routinely doing blood gas and hemoglobin tests in the air. The past limitations on mobile care delivery have been removed, and the medical profession must play catch-up to study and design proper utilization and quality control measures.

In summary, the current telemedicine marketplace, designed to send data from rural locations to distant specialists, has less value in an advanced urban or suburban home medical practice, where the provider makes decisions at the point of care. That said, there is a role for telemonitors in a home-based practice, with or without house calls. The author is saving his investment money for a telemonitor that is

1. Passively used to acquire data with minimal nuisance to the patient
2. Devoid of moving parts or maintenance needs
3. Capable of being sterilized or at least cleaned and reused
4. Designed to acquire physiologic signals, like impedance, instead of blood pressure
5. Capable of downloading patient instructions by Bluetooth or RF in the home
6. Capable of being a communication platform for appointments, trend line data, and information between collaborative providers making home visits
7. Available at slow upload speeds through a tablet computer wherever access can be gained to the Internet during travels
8. Capable of receiving passive wireless signals from digital sensors during a home visit; for example, having vital signs, oximetry, impedance, and digital x-rays insert automatically into the visit record.

SUMMARY

It must be said again that application of portable technology in advanced home care is an emerging field. It makes sense, and it is used daily by hundreds of practitioners, but it lacks a supporting evidence base. Many mobile clinicians, especially in a collaborative practice with home health nurses or their own mid-levels, have already become the leading high-tech providers in medicine today. Like the authors, they are convinced about the clinical efficacy and cost-saving potential of the paperless, wireless, and often keyboard-less practice.

Medicare reimbursement for home visits average around $100 without ancillaries, so making 10 home visits to prevent even a single $1,000 ambulance ride is cost-neutral for Medicare. Home medical care is only an added cost if it fails to offset acute care use. The government's demographic and financial pressure suggests a need to press ahead with the enhanced mobile care model, so the explosion in point-of-care devices should continue. The main challenge is to decide which ones provide dispositive value to patients.

REFERENCES

1. Lambe S, Washington DL, Fink A, et al. Waiting times in California's emergency departments. Ann Emerg Med 2003;41(1):35–44.
2. Leff B, Burton L, Mader SL, et al. Hospital at home: feasibility and outcomes of a program to provide hospital-level care at home for acutely ill older patients. Ann Intern Med 2005;143(11):798–808.
3. Bayne CG. Applying trans-thoracic impedance technologies in the diagnosis and monitoring of homebound CHF patients. Frontiers 2003;15(1):11–2.
4. EHR Exemption for HIT, Final Rule. Federal Register 71(152) on August 8, 2006.
5. The ONC-Coordinated Federal Health IT Strategic Plan 2008–2012. June 3, 2008.
6. Medicare Improvements for Patients and Providers Act of 2008, Section 132, signed by President Bush on June 24, 2008.
7. 42 CFR Part 423. Medicare Program; Medicare Part D Claims Data. Final Rule. May 23, 2008.

Workforce Development in Geriatric Home Care

Jennifer Hayashi, MD[a],*, Linda DeCherrie, MD[b], Edward Ratner, MD[c], Peter A. Boling, MD[d]

KEYWORDS

- Home health care • Home care • House calls
- Home care workforce • Geriatric workforce

Our nation is aging. Due to increases in life expectancy and aging of the baby boom generation, people older than 65 years made up 12% of the US population in 2005. By 2030, this percentage is predicted to grow to 20%. Although the majority maintains independent functioning and good health, three quarters have at least one chronic medical condition, and 20% of Medicare recipients have five or more chronic medical conditions.[1] Because the population is aging and most patients prefer to remain at home during periods of disability, the number of people who are temporarily or permanently homebound will increase rapidly. In 1998, 7.6 million persons received skilled home care services, and 69% were aged 65 years or older.[2] Although the proportion with disability may be slowly declining due to medical advances, the rapid increase in population size will produce a sharp rise in the absolute number of persons with disabilities.[3] More than 2 million persons, half of whom are older than 65 years, are permanently homebound according to Medicare criteria. For these patients, traveling to a medical office for routine or urgent care is difficult or impossible. Several million others need short-term home care when recovering from acute illnesses and injuries.

The focus of this article is on preparing the workforce needed for home-based care. Providing this care requires an extended team and many different types of workers. "Home care" is a broad term that includes diagnostic, therapeutic, or social support services provided in the home.[4] This includes skilled nursing, physical and occupational therapy, social support, and home health aide services, all provided by

[a] Johns Hopkins University School of Medicine, 5505 Hopkins Bayview Circle, Baltimore, MD 21224, USA
[b] Mount Sinai Medical Center, 1 Gustave L Levy Place, Box 1070, MMC 741, New York, NY 10029, USA
[c] University of Minnesota, 420 Delaware Street SE, Minneapolis, MN 55455,USA
[d] Virginia Commonwealth University, PO Box 980102, Richmond, VA 23298, USA
* Corresponding author.
E-mail address: jhayash1@jhmi.edu (J. Hayashi).

Clin Geriatr Med 25 (2009) 109–120
doi:10.1016/j.cger.2008.10.006
0749-0690/08/$ – see front matter © 2009 Elsevier Inc. All rights reserved.

Medicare-certified home health care agencies for persons who are Medicare-eligible. These services must be overseen by a physician. Home care also includes home medical care or house calls, which can be performed by a physician, nurse practitioner (NP), or physician assistant (PA). Community agencies also support patients in the home along with volunteers from programs such as Meals on Wheels, religious organizations, and friendly visitor programs. The vast majority of hands-on daily care is provided by paid personal care aides, most funded by Medicaid, and unpaid lay caregivers who carry the largest share of the daily care load. Merely maintaining, without improving, the current inadequate provider-patient ratio will require 3.5 million additional health care workers by 2030, a 35% increase.[1]

Physicians and other medical providers billed only 1.5 million home visits in 2002, which is less than one visit per year for every fifth or sixth skilled home care user. In contrast, similarly disabled, chronically ill nursing home patients are seen by a medical provider at their place of residence eight or nine times a year on average. The number of homebound older adults who could benefit from house calls is overwhelming in comparison to the number of qualified and willing providers.

Physicians who make house calls are mostly internists, geriatricians, and family physicians. Internal medicine residents have little or no training in house calls. The lack of training exposure to house calls is significant, because resident home visits are highly correlated with house calls in future practice.[4] Only about 25% of trainees in internal medicine have any exposure to providing or overseeing home care.[5] There is debate about how much home care teaching is needed in internal medicine residency and how this fits into already full schedules; yet the recent IOM report on the geriatric workforce recommends that hospitals encourage training of residents in all settings where older adults receive care, including nursing homes, assisted-living facilities, and patients' homes. This experience has also diminished in family medicine training; house calls are required, but in 2006, the requirement was reduced to two visits and emphasis placed on a more general requirement for competence in managing homebound patients. Geriatric fellows are required to have home care experience, and eventual enforcement of requirements for home care competency is anticipated; because most geriatric fellows come from internal medicine or family practice residencies, their current preparation for home care is limited. A recent survey of directors of academic geriatric programs concluded that geriatricians could provide the most benefit by focusing on the most complex and vulnerable older adults.[6]

There are some published examples of educational programs for medical students and residents that have made a positive impact on attitudes and knowledge regarding home care and house calls.[7–18] In general, these interventions increase trainees' self-reported awareness of systems-based practice, interdisciplinary teamwork, and empathy by giving them the opportunity to observe acute or chronic illness in the context of the rest of a patient's life. Some of these are grant-funded initiatives and may not be sustained over time, given other pressures on the curriculum and operational cost, but they support the view that this type of education is effective and practical.

Even if training for chronic care and home health care in residency was strong, few trainees are entering primary care specialties, especially geriatrics. As of 2007, only 7128 physicians are certified in geriatric medicine. According to the Alliance for Aging Research, 35,000 geriatricians will be needed by 2030.[1] There are 119 geriatric medicine fellowship programs, and in 2001-2002, there were 345 fellows in all years of geriatric fellowship training. Forty-six percent of the fellowship programs offered 1 year of training with a fill rate of 69%. Thirty-six percent of fellowship programs report no US medical school graduates as first year fellows.[19] In family medicine, there are 460 residency programs as of 2006, with 3527 interns and 9997 total residents. The number of programs and residents has increased over time, especially the number of residents, which has more than doubled since 1976. However, there were more than 10,000 residents in the late 1990s, and it is hard to predict the future.[20]

Paucity of home care education in medical school and residency may adversely affect the supply of physicians who can or will provide medical care to patients at home. There is no direct evidence that current interventions to increase home care education for physicians in training have resulted in a larger supply of geriatricians, but leading experts in geriatrics and health care policy[1,21,22] agree that educational interventions are a necessary component of the effort to meet the health care needs of America's aging population. With regard to curriculum content, **Table 1** shows some key elements that all physicians should master by the time of graduation from residency training if they are going to manage homebound patients with advanced chronic illness, and **Table 2** shows a curriculum outline for home health agency (HHA) medical directors, which is an expanding field for physicians in home care; the role parallels the medical director role now required in nursing homes and hospices.

Besides educational gaps, there are multiple other reasons why medical professionals, including physicians, choose specialties other than geriatrics, including ageism, lack of recognition by hospital and medical school leadership, low professional visibility of geriatrics in institutions, the challenging nature of chronic illness care, and Medicare reimbursement rates. Only 26.7% of physician income was derived from Medicare in 2000, whereas those who provide care to older adults obtain most of their clinical income from that source.[22]

Table 1
Core home care curricular components for graduating professionals

Interdisciplinary Teamwork	Medical Home Care
HHA care	When to make house calls
Patient selection/eligibility	No shows, cannot come in
Agency choice	Unexpected decline
Paperwork	Medical conditions refractory to usual
Team role (how to participate)	management
Medical equipment	Family request
Patient selection/eligibility	Acute care (triage criteria)
Oxygen	How to make house calls
Devices	Diagnostic technology
Paperwork	Charting (including HER)
Specialty care	Home assessment
IV therapy	Home as unique setting
Ventilators	Patient's turf (guest status)
Artificial feeding	Social dimensions
Catheters	Caregiver assessment/support
Wounds	Billing for services
Telemedicine	House calls
Monitoring systems	Domiciliary care
Virtual visits	Care plan oversight
Evidence base	Care certification
Outcome studies in home care	

Abbreviations: HER, health record; HHA, home health agency; IV, intravenous.

Table 2 Core curriculum for home health agency medical director	
Administrative oversight of HHA patient care process	HHA rules and regulations Denials and appeals process Survey process Stark regulations Fraud and abuse
Community liaison	Physician education Helping the difficult physician Developing advisory panels
Ethics, patient advocacy	Under-service and discriminatory selection Serving the "difficult" patient Evaluating unusual service requests Closing unsafe/inappropriate cases
Quality improvement	OASIS and OBQI Other approaches (P-D-C-A, etc)
HHA staff education	In-services and one-one
Job description, contracting	Defining your role Creating legal medical director contracts
HHA culture and finance	Medicare PPS reimbursement Other contracts Use review
Employee health	Screening OSHA Episodic illness
Research	IRB-approved clinical studies

Abbreviations: HHA, home health agency; IRB, Institutional Review Board; OASIS, Outcome Assessment and Information Set; OBQI, outcomes-based quality improvement; OSHA, Occupational Safety and Health Administration; P-D-C-A, plan, do, check, act; PPS, prospective payment system.

Data from American Academy of Home Care Physicians. Medical directorship of home health agencies: a brief guide to physician administration in the realm of the home health industry. Edgewood, MD; AAHCP, 2008.

However, there are also many reasons for people choosing careers in geriatrics, including altruism, perceived societal need for geriatric care, the nonmedical aspects of the specialty, and the range of medical problems addressed by geriatricians. On another positive note, geriatricians generally rate career satisfaction higher than physicians do in any other medical specialty.[23]

In the end, poor financial opportunities may discourage students with high educational debt from choosing careers in geriatrics and may lead to practicing physicians leaving the field. A recent analysis of financial return on the educational investment for internists with certification in geriatrics showed that geriatricians' incomes were consistently lower than those of general internists over the 7-year period from 1993 to 1997, although the disparity varied from 27% in 1993 to 9% in 1997 and remained stable at 10% by 1999.[24] Income expectation and perceived professional status, a closely related factor, are strong predictors of specialty choice among medical students.[25] Better financial and other incentives are needed to generate a robust geriatric workforce, and this requires a change in health policy; the new policy approach must produce a system that pays for services that add the most societal value and also contribute to controlling the current unsustainable rate of rise in health care costs, as articulated by McClellan, a noted health economist and prior administrator for the Medicare and Medicaid programs.[26] Current incentives favor increased volumes of high-technology procedures, inpatient care, and specialized medical services, not care coordination and comprehensive care of patients with complex problems.

Improving reimbursement for direct care, while necessary, is only one form of financial incentive. Other strategies have been shown effective in meeting health care needs of underserved populations: scholarships, loan repayment, direct financial incentives, and service-option loans provide financial assistance to students and residents in return for obligated service periods. In general, such programs lead to more care for the target population, longer physician service in high-need areas, and higher physician satisfaction, with 90% of obligated physicians reporting that they would enroll in such programs again if they had the opportunity.[27] These promising results suggest that similar incentives, if applied to geriatrics training and home care, might attract and retain physicians in the field. Again, geriatrics and policy experts agree that these incentives are part of a multifactorial approach to grow the physician workforce for the next half century.

NPs and PAs are non-physician clinicians who are playing an increasingly important role in care for the elderly, although the number of these clinicians making home visits remains small, and in 2002 only about 4% of NPs were certified geriatric NPs. In 2004, the American Association of Colleges of Nursing with a grant from the Hartford foundation created NP and clinical nurse specialist competencies in older adult care, realizing that most of these trainees do not go into geriatrics but all will care for older adults. These competencies are thorough but do not specifically mention home care or any site-specific training.[28] We could find no information about the extent to which these professionals have home care experience during training. Though NP training competencies do not specify home care experience, they do explicitly recognize that gerontological NPs work in a variety of settings, including the patient's home.[29]

Similarly, according to a 2004 survey of the American Academy of Physician Assistants (AAPA), only 185 members (0.6%) identified geriatrics as their primary specialty, whereas 130 of respondents (80.2%) reported that their work location was a nursing home or other long-term care facility. No information was provided about medical house calls to older patients.[30] PA school accreditation standards require clinical experience in outpatient, inpatient, emergency room, operating room, and long-term care, but we found no mention of home care education or experience.[31] The scant evidence base for the education and employment of these practitioners precludes in-depth analysis of effective remedies for their portion of the workforce shortage in home care. Although the same factors influencing the physician workforce may pertain, another barrier may be the lack of on-site professional support and supervision in the home setting compared with other sites.

The AAHCP, which has a growing number of NP and PA members, has led many of the efforts to expand training in home care medicine. Its continuing education courses, faculty development programs, publications, multimedia materials, and certification exams in home care medicine and home care medical direction offer learning opportunities and validation. These should help those educators seeking to teach this content. Considerable growth in interest is still needed to expand the number of AAHCP-certified providers from the currently modest 150.

Data on geriatric and home care content in curricula for professional nursing, physical therapy, occupational therapy, and social work are less widely available than data on physician geriatric training. However, similar shortages of adequately prepared clinicians exist in all of these disciplines. For example, less than 1% of 2.2 million practicing nurses have gerontological certification. Baccalaureate programs, which provide approximately one-third of all registered nurse (RN) degrees, generally lack sufficient full-time faculty certified in geriatrics and have little or no formal geriatric content, such as geriatric courses or geriatric clinical training sites.[2] Nursing faces a critical staffing shortage both in general and in geriatrics. According to the US Bureau of Labor Statistics in 2006, 126,453 (5%) of 2,504,664 US nurses were employed byHHAs, yet many graduated from nursing school with minimal geriatric training. This large, experienced workforce is vital to the future of home care but may have some specific educational needs.

Therapists are also able to specialize in geriatrics, but less than 0.3% of physical therapists are certified "geriatric clinical specialists."[32] Although about 50% of speech and language pathology (SLP) therapists work with the elderly, mostly in institutional settings, no information was found regarding their geriatric or home care training. According to the US Department of Labor, there will be an 11% increase in the need for SLP between 2006 and 2016. For occupational therapists, there will be a 23% increase in need over the same interval, and as in the other disciplines, there are no data on training specific to home care or geriatric care.

Social work also reports inadequate numbers of geriatric workers. Although the numbers are harder to quantify, less than 3% reported majors in aging or gerontological social work,[2] and only 5% identify their primary practice area as geriatrics.[22] Most social workers receive little or no formal training in working with homebound elderly.

Due to insufficient formal training in geriatrics for these professionals, private organizations, such as the John A. Hartford Foundation, have funded academic mentoring programs in nursing and social work, with positive results but small overall increases in numbers of academic leaders in these fields.[33–35] No generalizable information is available about financial incentives for allied health professionals, although it has been noted that a 2007 survey of practicing RNs revealed that RNs practicing in geriatrics had the lowest hourly wages among 14 types of settings.[36] The federal government, through the Bureau of Health Professions, funds 41 state-level Geriatric Education Centers (GECs), which focus on training for practicing professionals and educators. A clearinghouse of more than 1100 GEC educational materials has only seven items related to home care.

The direct care workforce (home health and personal care aides) and family caregivers are the front line in keeping patients at home, although they receive little or no training. The number of persons needing the services of a caregiver is expected to more than double from 13 million in 2000 to 27 million in 2050,[37] whereas the number of "potential" caregivers aged 50 to 64 years will decrease from 21 (in 1970) to six (in 2030) per elderly patient.[38] There is a current and predicted severe shortage of paid caregivers, and most of these individuals have little formal training in elder care. Overall, their work is poorly paid and underappreciated.

While Newcomer and Stone (see the article elsewhere in this issue) address these and other challenges facing direct care workers, the importance of these workers in home care warrants additional attention here. The number of workers providing this type of care in noninstitutional care settings tripled between 1989 and 2004, which parallels expansion in Medicaid funding for it. These workers have the poorest retention rates of all health care workers, compounding the recruitment problem common to all fields. They must overcome many of the same challenges as their professional counterparts, including inadequate training and low wages compared with other job choices.[39] They also face barriers in the form of low education levels, lower socioeconomic status, racial discrimination, and other employment issues, such as lack of health insurance and absence of organized advocacy.[37,40] In particular, home care aides and attendants work with individual patients without accessible collegial support systems. Several national organizations, including the IOM, the US Department of Health and Human Services, and the US General Accounting Office, have called attention to the widening gap between supply and demand of these essential care providers.

Extensive research by the nonprofit Paraprofessional Healthcare Institute indicates that improvements in wages, benefits, training, organizational culture, and career development opportunities have clear, positive effects on outcomes, such as worker retention and job satisfaction, in a variety of long-term care settings, including patients' homes.[41] Although long-range national policy solutions remain elusive, there is mounting evidence that state-level interventions, such as California's Caregiver Training Initiative, that target these barriers can achieve measurable and sustainable gains in the geriatric direct care workforce.

The most numerous and, arguably, most important in home caregivers are family members, friends, and neighbors. Commonly called informal caregivers, they provide live-in or intermittent help on an unpaid basis. Over three-quarters (78%) of adults receiving long-term care at home rely exclusively on informal caregiving.[42] The workload is staggering. In the United States, it is estimated that more than 50 million individuals provide such care to an ill or disabled adult.[43] Although about half of caregivers provide fewer than 8 hours of care per week, nearly 1 in 5 provide at least the equivalent of full-time care (40 hours per week or more).[44] In 1997, the cost of replacing these services with paid care was estimated at $196 billion, which was approximately twice the combined spending for HHA ($32 billion) and nursing home services ($83 billion).[45]

Compared with formal caregiving, provided by paid individuals who typically have no prior relationship with the person requiring home care, informal care has 2 main advantages. First, informal caregiving is generally consistent over time. In 2003, the National Alliance for Caregiving and American Association of Retired Persons (AARP) surveyed current informal caregivers and found that they (usually a child or spouse) had been providing that care for an average of 4.3 years.[46] Over such extended periods, the need for paid caregivers to share cases and staff turnover would potentially require dozens of individuals to learn the client's care needs. The second advantage of informal caregiving is the level of emotional investment. Informal caregivers and care recipients nearly always have had mutually meaningful relationships before and possibly during care. This often produces levels of commitment to caregiving not possible in the formal caregiving system.

The benefits of informal caregiving are notable. Careful statistical analysis of a nationally representative sample of nearly 7000 elderly patients found that informal caregiving in the home is associated with a lower risk of nursing home admission,[47] although this was not confirmed in a study of the frail and very poor population enrolled in Program of All-Inclusive Care for the Elderly (PACE).[48] In contrast, PACE participants with a spouse as a caregiver had significantly reduced mortality.[49]

The burdens on informal caregivers have been well documented and include harm to both physical and mental health together with significant financial burden. These caregivers are often under major financial pressures and personal stress and have poorer health, more depression, and less social interaction than noncaregivers.[50] Increased blood pressure and insulin levels, impaired immune systems, and increased risk for cardiovascular disease have been shown.[51] Depression has been found in 20% to 50% of caregivers, with the highest rates among those providing dementia-related care. Those who care for persons with long-term chronic illness are more likely to die during the process than other caregivers.[52] Caregivers are estimated to have losses of income over their lifetime of about $700,000.[53]

Given the vital importance of this workforce, it is essential to support them. Health care and social services systems support informal caregivers in several ways. Many organizations provide information and referral to help caregivers find formal support.

A vital source is government-supported Area Agencies on Aging, and numerous websites now provide links to community services. There are limited governmental or charitable financial supports for informal caregivers, but little progress has been made with efforts to expand tax credits or offer adult caregivers time off from work, a benefit that is available for childcare. Some state Medicaid systems allow family caregivers to receive payment for providing covered personal care services. Caregiver training and coaching are increasingly common. Finally, bereavement support, routinely in hospice programs, helps those who have struggled with caregiving to the end of life.

Outside of hospice, the issues and needs of informal caregivers have been relatively disregarded by medical care providers, whose focus is on the patient. Yet, the informal caregiver is often the key to success of the medical care plan, and thus they deserve attention. Communication with at least one informal caregiver should be a routine part of many, if not all, medical encounters involving frail older persons, to identify issues not raised by the patient and to negotiate changes to the care plan. For example, when a medication change is planned, the prescriber should consider discussing this with someone involved with obtaining the prescription, setting up or dispensing it, and monitoring its effects. Primary care providers should help informal caregivers find needed formal support services, even if only recommending reliable information and referral programs. Finally, primary care providers should recognize end-of-life scenarios and suggest hospice care. After death, primary care providers can bring closure to relationships with informal caregivers by recognizing bereavement, at least with a condolence card.

Volunteers in public and private organizations provide an unmeasured amount of care to older adults at home, through formal programs such as Meals on Wheels and friendly visitor services as well as informal assistance with shopping, banking, and other errands. The extent and varied modes of care in this service network have not been quantified, but results from an innovative program in North Carolina suggest that older adult volunteers can provide important assistance. The Experience Corps for Independent Living (ECIL) recruited volunteers older than 55 years to expand the scope of independent living services for frail older people and their caregivers in specific communities, through 6 different demonstration projects over 3 years. ECIL was particularly successful in providing independent living services to frail elders and their families but was less successful in achieving the outcome of a cohesive, self-supporting team and failed to attract and retain the anticipated number of volunteers during the study period.[54]

In the end, many of the factors that lead people to work in home care are intangible and difficult to measure. For lay caregivers, these likely include family attachments and duty. For paid workers, aspects such as variety in daily experience, freedom from the constraints of office or institutional care settings, "making a difference," gratitude from those that receive care, opportunities to solve problems creatively, and missionary spirit all may contribute.

SUMMARY

The US population, with its increasing life expectancy and disability burden, faces a steadily worsening shortage of geriatric health care workers and informal caregivers. As the population grows older and sicker, increasing functional impairment and dependency will intensify the need for motivated and trained home care providers. Although there is a limited evidence base to forecast the best strategies for remedying the shortage and averting this impending health care crisis, the data summarized here suggest several crucial elements that must be addressed.

First, geriatric education of professional providers and lay caregivers must be promoted and improved, with special attention to the knowledge, attitudes, and skills needed to care for medically complex older patients at home. There is a key educational agenda related to coordinated, advanced chronic illness care, and many experts now think that it should be funded at least in substantial part by government and tied to payment for care.[55]

Second, compensation for the currently undervalued work of caring for older patients must be brought up to a level comparable to that of other fields, not only directly through equitable reimbursement but also indirectly through loan repayment and other systematic incentives across disciplines and with respect to informal caregivers. These 2 central interventions, finance and education reform, are ultimately intertwined and must occur simultaneously. Certainly, funding will beget training, if there is a strong interest in entering the field.

Finally, in a broad sense, the art and science of caring for older adults at home must become widely recognized as challenging, rewarding, and socially valuable to attract and retain qualified professionals and aides. Safe and effective coordination of care over time and across settings from the acute care hospital through subacute care to home must be valued as highly as the latest technological breakthroughs. The future of our health care system and our nation depends on it.

REFERENCES

1. Committe on the Future Health Care Workforce for Older Americans. Retooling for an Aging America: Building the Health Care Workforce. Washington, DC; Institute of Medicine; 2008.
2. Kovner CT, Mezey M, Harrington C. Who cares for older adults? Workforce implications of an aging society. Health Aff 2002;21:78–89.
3. Rice DP, Fineman N. Economic implications of increased longevity in the United States. Annu Rev Public Health 2004;25:457–73.
4. Levine SA, Boal J, Boling PA. Home care. JAMA 2003;290(9):1203–7.
5. Stoltz CM, Smith LG, Boal JH. Home care training in internal medicine residencies: a national survey. Acad Med 2001;76:181–3.
6. Warshaw G, Bragg EJ, Fried LP, et al. Which patients benefit the most from a geriatrician's care? Consensus among directors of geriatrics academic programs. J Am Geriatr Soc 2008;56:1796–801.
7. Matter CA, Speice JA, McCann R, et al. Hospital to home: Improving internal medicine residents' understanding of the needs of older persons after a hospital stay. Acad Med 2003;78(8):793–7.
8. Duque G, Fung S, Mallet L, et al. Learning while having fun: the use of video gaming to teach geriatric house calls to medical students. J Am Geriatr Soc 2008; 56(7):1328–32.
9. Lai CJ, Nye HE, Bookwalter T, et al. Postdischarge follow-up visits for medical and pharmacy students on an inpatient medicine clerkship. J Hosp Med 2008;3(1): 20–7.
10. Hervada-Page M, Favock KS, Sifri R, et al. The home visit experience: a medical student's perspective. Care Manag J 2007;8(4):206–10.
11. McWilliams A, Rosemond C, Roberts E, et al. An innovative home-based interdisciplinary service-learning experience. Gerontol Geriatr Educ 2008;28(3):89–104.
12. Boling PA, Willett RM, Gentili A, et al. The importance of "high valence" events in a successful program for teaching geriatrics to medical students. Gerontol Geriatr Educ 2008;28(3):59–72.

13. Hayashi JL, Phillips KA, Arbaje A, et al. A curriculum to teach internal medicine residents to perform house calls for older adults. J Am Geriatr Soc 2007;55(8): 1287–94.

14. Wheeler BK, Powelson S, Kim JH. Interdisciplinary clinical education: implementing a gerontological home visiting program. Nurse Educ 2007;32(3):136–40.

15. Lee M, Kaufman A. The University of New Mexico visiting physicians program: helping older New Mexicans stay at home. Care Manag J 2006;7(1):45–50.

16. Yuen JK, Breckman R, Adelman RD, et al. Reflections of medical students on visiting chronically ill older patients in the home. J Am Geriatr Soc 2006;54(11): 1778–83.

17. Laditka SB, Fischer M, Mathews KB, et al. There's no place like home: evaluating family medicine residents' training in home care. Home Health Care Serv Q 2002;21(2):1–17.

18. Medina-Walpole A, Heppard B, Clark NS, et al. Mi Casa o Su Casa? Assessing function and values in the home. J Am Geriatr Soc 2005;53(2):336–42.

19. Beck JC, Butler RN. Physician recruitment into geriatrics: further insight into the black box. J Am Geriatr Soc 2004;52:1959–61.

20. Available at: http://www.aafp.org/online/en/home/aboutus/specialty/facts/20.html. Accessed October 5, 2008.

21. Association of Directors of Geriatric Academic Programs Website. Available at: http://www.adgapstudy.uc.edu/Home.cfm. Accessed July 15, 2008.

22. Lamascus AM, Bernard MA, Barry P, et al. Bridging the workforce gap for our aging society: how to increase and improve knowledge and training. Report of an expert panel. J Am Geriatr Soc 2005;53:343–7.

23. Leigh JP, Kravitz RL, Schembri M, et al. Physician career satisfaction across specialties. Arch Intern Med 2002;162:1577–84.

24. Weeks WB, Wallace AE. Return on educational investment in geriatrics training. J Am Geriatr Soc 2004;52:1940–5.

25. Reed VA, Jernstedt GC, Reber ES. Understanding and improving medical student specialty choice: a synthesis of the literature using decision theory as a referent. Teach Learn Med 2001;13:117–29.

26. McClellan MB. Rising to the challenge of real health care reform. Brookings Institution, 2008. Available at: http://www.brookings.edu/opinions/2008/10_health_reform_mcclellan.aspx. Accessed October 19, 2008.

27. Pathman DE, Konrad TR, King TS, et al. Outcomes of states' scholarships, loan repayment, and related programs for physicians. Med Care 2004;42:560–8.

28. Nurse practitioner and clinical nurse specialist competencies for older adult care, March 2004. Available at: http://www.aacn.nche.edu/Education/pdf/APNCompetencies.pdf. Accessed October 5, 2008.

29. National Organization of Nurse Practitioner Faculties; in partnership with American Association of Colleges of Nursing. Nurse Practitioner Primary Care Competencies in Specialty Areas. Adult, Family, Gerontological, Pediatric, and Women's Health. Rockville (MD); Department of Health and Human Services, Health Care Resources and Services Administration. Available at: http://www.aanp.org/NR/rdonlyres/E1B37354-2195-401D-8027-A5A2763E3006/0/finalaug2002.pdf. Accessed October 5, 2008.

30. Brugna RA. The physician assistant role in geriatric medicine and rehabilitation. Phys Occup Ther Geriatr 2006;25:67–76.

31. Accreditation Standards for Physician Assistant Education by the Accreditation Review. Commission on education for physician assistants October 2007. Available at: http://www.arc-pa.org/Standards/3rdeditionwithPDchangesandregionals4.24.08a.pdf.

32. American Academy of Physician Assistants. Available at: http://www.AAPA.org. Accessed July 15, 2008.
33. Berman A, Mezey M, Kobayashi M, et al. Gerontological nursing content in baccalaureate nursing programs: comparison of findings from 1997 and 2003. J Prof Nurs 2005;21:268–75.
34. Maas ML, Strumptf NE, Beck C, et al. Mentoring geriatric nurse scientists, educators, clinicians, and leaders in the John A. Hartford foundation centers for geriatric nursing excellence. Nurs Outlook 2006;54:183–8.
35. Mackin LA, Kayser-Jones J, Franklin PD, et al. Successful recruiting into geriatric nursing: the experience of the John A. Hartford foundation centers of geriatric nursing excellence. Nurs Outlook 2006;54:197–203.
36. Ericksen AB. 2007 Earnings survey. RN 2007;70:42–8.
37. Kaye HS, Chapman S, Newcomer RJ, et al. The personal assistance workforce: trends in supply and demand. Health Aff 2006;25:1113–20.
38. Chronic Care in America: A 21st Century Challenge. Princeton (NJ): Robert Wood Johnson Foundation; 1996. p. 76.
39. Matthias R, Morrison E, Chapman S, et al. Caregiver training initiative process and implementation evaluation. Los Angeles: California Employment Development Department; 2002.
40. Neysmith SM, Aronson J. Working conditions in home care: negotiating race and class boundaries in gendered work. Int J Health Serv 1997;27:479–99.
41. Dawson S. Recruitment and retention of paraprofessionals. In: Paraprofessional Health Institute presentation to Institute of Medicine, June 28, 2007. Available at: www.directclearinghouse.org. Accessed July 30, 2008.
42. Thompson L. Long-term care: support for family caregivers. Long-Term Care Financing Project, Issues Brief. Georgetown University; March 2004.
43. Health and Human Services. Informal Caregiving: Compassion in Action. Based on data from the National Survey of Families and Households (NSFH). Washington, DC: Department of Health and Human Services; 1998.
44. Alzheimer's Association and National Alliance for Caregiving. Families care: Alzheimer's caregiving in the United States. Chicago (IL): Alzheimer's Association; 2004. Bethesda (MD): National Alliance for Caregiving.
45. Arno PS, Levine C, Memmott M. The economic value of informal caregiving. Health Aff 1999;18:182–8.
46. National Alliance for Caregiving and AARP. Caregiving in the U.S. Bethesda (MD): National Alliance for Caregiving; 2004. Washington DC: AARP.
47. Charles KK, Sevak P. Can family caregiving substitute for nursing home care? J Health Econ 2005;24:1174–90.
48. Friedman SM, Steinwachs DM, Temkin-Greener H, et al. Informal caregivers and the risk of nursing home admission among individuals enrolled in the program of all-inclusive care for the elderly. Gerontologist 2006;46:456–63.
49. Temkin-Greener H, Bajorska A, Peterson DR, et al. Social support and risk-adjusted mortality in a frail older population. Med Care 2004;42:779–88.
50. Haley WF, Levine EG, Brown SL, et al. Psychological, social, and health consequences of caring for a relative with senile dementia. J Am Geriatr Soc 1987; 35:405–11.
51. Schulz R, Beach SR. Caregiving as a risk factor for mortality: the caregiver health effects study. JAMA 1999;282(23):2215–9.
52. Christakis NA, Allison PD. Mortality after the hospitalization of a spouse. N Engl J Med 2006;354(7):719–30.

53. Family Caregiver Alliance. Selected Caregiver Statistics Fact Sheet. Available at: http://www.caregiver.org/caregiver/jsp/content_node.jsp?nodeid=439&;expandnodeid=480. Accessed July 27, 2008.

54. Rabiner DJ, Koetse EC, Nemo B. An overview and critique of the Experience Corps for Independent Living initiative. J Aging Soc Policy 2003;15:55–78.

55. Iglehart JK. Medicare, graduate medical education, and new policy directions. N Engl J Med 2008;359(6):643–50.

The History of Quality Measurement in Home Health Care

Robert J. Rosati, PhD

KEYWORDS

- Home health care • Quality improvement • OASIS
- OBQI • QIO

There is little debate that focusing on quality improvement can result in improved patient outcomes and reduce the cost of health care delivery. Home health care is no different from other sectors of the delivery system in its need to focus on improving quality. This article provides a perspective on the current state of quality improvement, how it has evolved, and where it is headed.

OASIS DEVELOPMENT AND IMPLEMENTATION

Understanding the impact of care delivery and, therefore, its quality requires the measurement of patient outcomes to assess both intended and unintended effects. Home health care is in a unique position, measuring health status when patients enter and exit care, allowing evaluation of individual patient outcomes. In 1995, Shaughnessy and colleagues[1] proposed that a new assessment tool could become the basis of outcome based quality improvement (OBQI). The tool was called Outcome and Assessment Information Set (OASIS). An early form of OASIS was released in 1994 after 5 years of research conducted by the Center for Health Services Research and Policy at the University of Colorado.[2] Because a wide variety of factors influence home care outcomes, OASIS includes items related to demographics and patient history, supportive assistance, sensory status, integumentary status, respiratory status, elimination status, neurological/emotional/behavioral status, activities of daily living (ADLs), instrumental activities of daily living, ability to manage medications, equipment management, emergent care (EC), and discharge disposition. The instrument contains nearly 100 items that cover all of these domains, and because patients' condition changes rapidly in home care, OASIS was designed to be collected at admission or resumption of care, follow-up time points (every 60 days), and at transfer or discharge.

Changes in scores from start of care to discharge allow for the computation of patient outcomes. In October 2000, the Centers for Medicare and Medicaid Services

Centre for Home Care Policy & Research, Visiting Nurse Service of New York, 1250 Broadway, 20th Floor, New York, NY 10001, USA
E-mail address: robert.rosati@vnsny.org

Clin Geriatr Med 25 (2009) 121–134
doi:10.1016/j.cger.2008.11.001
0749-0690/08/$ – see front matter © 2009 Elsevier Inc. All rights reserved.

(CMS) mandated that OASIS be collected on all Medicare and Medicaid patients receiving skilled services. The current version of OASIS-B1, which is based on revisions made in 2002[3] and 2008, is available on the CMS Web site (http://www.cms.hhs.gov/oasis/). Since its inception, there has been debate about the value of OASIS within the home health care industry. Questions have been raised about the reliability of the instrument,[4–6] burden of completing the assessment due to the length, and value as an indicator of quality.[7] Nonetheless, OASIS seems to have survived the controversy and become a fundamental component of home health care quality assessment. Some organizations have shown that OASIS is a tool to improve quality,[8] and the industry, in general, has begun to rely on it as a major component of quality improvement efforts.[9]

RISK ADJUSTMENT

To level the playing field and address provider concerns that their outcomes are worse "because our patients are sicker," a fundamental component of being able to accurately assess outcomes across providers is the ability to risk adjust measures based on patient characteristics. From the early development of OASIS, consideration was given to developing case mix or risk-adjusted outcome measures. Patient outcomes are adjusted based on start or resumption of care assessment information. For example, a statistical model was developed to risk adjust the improvement in dressing the lower body based on whether the patient lives alone, receives assistance provided by a caregiver, level of functional status at start of care, and the presence of other specific clinical conditions (eg, The International Classification of Diseases, Ninth Revision (ICD-9) diagnoses).[10] All 41 outcomes that can be generated from OASIS have separate risk-adjustment models. Each model includes a large number of variables, yet the models vary in the amount of explained variance from 10% to 27%. The measures are valid and statistically significant, but the unexplained variance highlights the challenge of outcome measurement in the home setting. CMS provides patient outcome reports to home health care agencies based on the risk-adjusted models. In late 2008, CMS released a new set of risk-adjustment models that will take into account recent changes in the characteristics of the home health care population.

PROSPECTIVE PAYMENT SYSTEM

One of the unexpected uses of OASIS was the mandate to base per-episode Medicare home health care reimbursement on how patients scored on the assessment at start of care. In 2000, there was a shift from cost-based fee-for-service reimbursement to prospective lump-sum payment for 60-day episodes of care.[11] Selected items from OASIS are used to assign severity scores in three domains: clinical, functional, and service use.

The clinical and service use domains have four levels of severity: minimal, low, moderate, and high. The functional status domain adds an additional level called maximum. Levels are determined based on a complicated scoring system, and reimbursement increases when the three domains are scored higher. The clinical domain is based on ICD-9 diagnoses, vision impairment, reported pain, treatment for wounds, shortness of breath, urinary and/or bowel incontinence, bowel ostomy, and behavioral problems. The functional domain includes the level of impairment in dressing, bathing, toileting, and locomotion.

The service use domain is based on whether the patient was admitted from the community or came from a rehabilitation or skilled nursing facility and whether the patient is expected to receive physical or occupational therapy visits during the home care episode. The initial therapy visit criterion was a threshold of at least

10 visits: above nine visits resulted in higher payment, and there was no further adjust-ment if more than 10 therapy visits were rendered. Scores on the three domains put patients into one of 80 Home Health Resource Groups (HHRGs), which determine re-imbursement for the episode of care. HHRGs are similar in concept to diagnostic re-lated groups used for hospital reimbursement.

In 2008, there was a major revision of Prospective Payment System (PPS), with ad-justments for early versus late episodes if patients remain open for extended periods (adjustment applies for the third or later contiguous 60-day episodes for a patient) and the amount of therapy services provided to a patient.[12] Therefore, reimbursement in-creases the longer the patient is in care (>120 days). The therapy domain now includes two thresholds of 14 and 20 visits, addressing higher severity levels. The functional do-main did not change substantially, but the clinical domain now includes several addi-tional diagnoses and combinations of diagnoses that are known to drive cost of care (eg, diabetes and renal failure). The new PPS has 153 HHRGs, with higher reimburse-ment for patients needing therapy and remaining in home health care for extended episodes of care. The range in an average payment from the top categories (~$8,000) to the bottom (~$2,000) is substantial.

OUTCOME-BASED QUALITY IMPROVEMENT

The capability to derive risk-adjusted outcomes allows health care organizations to compare themselves to national benchmarks to determine whether patients are re-ceiving optimal care. It also allows payers, regulators, and consumers to determine the quality of care provided by an organization. During the development and testing of OASIS, the concept of OBQI was created to describe the use of OASIS in organi-zational improvement. This was integrated into the rollout of OASIS across the home care industry but also coincided with a period of financial stress under the In-terim Payment System (1997–2000), during which agencies lost staff and drastically cut their education budgets, which probably delayed the impact on improving the quality of care.

OBQI outcome reports were designed for agencies to compare their functional, health, and utilization outcomes to national averages and determine areas for im-provement.[1] Functional and health outcomes are typically reported as the percentage of patients who are stabilized or improved. For example, there are measures such as stabilization in transferring and improvement in transferring. It is important to have measures that capture stabilization (no decline) rather than improvement for certain patient groups in which improvement is not likely. Examples of health outcomes in-clude measures of stabilization or improvement in pain interfering with activity, dysp-nea, depression, and confusion. An important measure of utilization is the rate of acute care hospitalizations within the first 60 days of care.

There are currently 30 OBQI measures, shown in **Table 1**, that an agency can use to assess the quality of the care being delivered and identify opportunities to design im-provement projects. For example, high rates of acute care hospitalizations may indi-cate poor communications with the physician, lack of patient compliance with taking medication, or failure to rapidly identify high-risk patients so that they receive more focused attention early in the episode. The OBQI measures have also been used to drive quality improvement initiatives at a national level.

OUTCOME-BASED QUALITY MANAGEMENT

In 2001, CMS introduced a new set of quality outcomes referred to as Outcome-Based Quality Management (OBQM) measures.[13] The measures are meant to represent

Table 1
Home health quality measures (outcome-based quality improvement outcomes)

End-result outcomes

Improvement in grooming

Stabilization in grooming

Improvement in upper body dressing

Improvement in lower body dressing

Improvement in bathing

Stabilization in bathing

Improvement in toileting

Improvement in transferring

Stabilization in transferring

Improvement in ambulation/locomotion

Improvement in eating

Improvement in light meal preparation

Stabilization in light meal preparation

Improvement in laundry

Stabilization in laundry

Improvement in housekeeping

Stabilization in housekeeping

Improvement in shopping

Stabilization in shopping

Improvement in phone use

Stabilization in phone use

Improvement in management of oral medications

Stabilization in management of oral medications

Improvement in dyspnea

Improvement in urinary tract infection

Improvement in urinary incontinence

Improvement in bowel incontinence

Improvement in pain interfering with activity

Improvement in number of surgical wounds

Improvement in status of surgical wounds

Improvement in speech and language

Stabilization in speech and language

Improvement in confusion frequency

Improvement in cognitive functioning

Stabilization in cognitive functioning

Improvement in anxiety level

Stabilization in anxiety level

Improvement in behavior problem frequency

Utilization outcomes

Discharged to community

Acute care hospitalization (lower values preferred)

Any EC (lower values preferred)

Abbreviation: EC, emergent care.

infrequent untoward or adverse events. Adverse events identified by these measures are thought to be markers for potential problems in care delivery. It is important to emphasize the word "potential" in this definition, because adverse events may not occur due to the care delivered but could be naturally occurring events. Whether or not an individual patient's poor outcome results from inadequate care can only be determined through review of the care delivered to the patient.

There are 13 adverse event measures that fall into four categories: EC, significant decline in health or function, significant unmet care needs, and serious unexpected events. **Table 2** shows the measures in each category. These are difficult measures for home health care agencies to use for quality improvement. First, they are extremely low-frequency events; most occur in less than 1% of episodes. Most agencies do not have enough patients with an adverse event to identify a meaningful trend that indicates a need to change practice. Second, the measures are not risk adjusted; therefore, it becomes impossible to make comparisons across organizations. Third, some measures (eg, unexpected death) have been criticized, because they are based on life expectancy of more than 6 months estimated at the start of care and are reported at a point when the patient's clinical condition might have changed. Nonetheless, these measures have remained, and one is now publicly reported: EC for wound infection or deteriorating wound status.

PUBLIC REPORTING

Public reporting of quality outcomes began in the early 1990s with hospitals and was expanded to nursing homes, dialysis facilities, and physicians in the last few years. In late 2003, CMS started to publicly report on 11 OBQI outcomes. CMS launched Home Health Compare on the Medicare.gov Web site and ran advertisements in local newspapers that information about individual agencies was available online. The goal was

Table 2
Adverse event measures (outcome-based quality management)
EC events
EC for injury caused by fall or accident at home
EC for wound infection or deteriorating wound status
EC for improper medication administration or medication side effects
EC for hypo/hyperglycemia
Significant decline in health or function
Development of urinary tract infection
Increase in number of pressure ulcers
Substantial decline in 3 or more ADLs
Substantial decline in management of medications
Significant unmet care need
Unmet need for wound care or medication assistance
Unmet need for toileting assistance
Unmet need for management of behavioral problem
Serious unexpected event
Unexpected nursing home admission
Unexpected death

Abbreviations: ADLs, activities of daily living; EC, emergent care.

to provide information to consumers so that they could choose an agency with the best outcomes in their geographic area. The measures reported were the same risk adjusted outcomes that agencies have been receiving in reports from CMS since 2001. The only difference between the publicly reported measures and those provided to the agencies was the labeling of the outcomes. "Improvement in ambulation and locomotion" was changed to "percentage of patients who get better at walking and moving around" on the CMS Web site. In 2007, an OBQM adverse event measure was added to Home Health Compare. Beyond patients using Home Health Compare, it is also possible for discharge planners, social workers, and physicians to use the reports when referring to home health care. To date, there are no reported data that show that this information is used by patients or providers.

PAY FOR PERFORMANCE

The initiative to increase reimbursement for high-quality care and reduce payment for low-performing hospitals and physicians has already started. Sometime in the near future, pay for performance will influence home health care. In a report to Congress in 2005, the Medicare Payment Advisory Commission (MedPAC) stated:

"Home health care has a ready set of outcomes measures that are already collected and have good risk adjustment. Outcome measures from CMS's Outcome-Based Quality Indicators set could form the starter set of pay-for-performance measures. The National Quality Forum, Agency for Healthcare Research and Quality (AHRQ), and an expert panel convened by CMS concur that a set of these measures are reliable and adequately risk adjusted. They pose no additional data collection burden because they have been collected and computed by home health agencies and CMS since 1999. Risk adjustment is supported by data on patient prognosis, functional status at the start and completion of care, multiple diagnoses, and behavioral and cognitive status."[14]

The report suggested that more work was needed to develop measures related to adverse events, such as falls in the home or potentially dangerous dehydration. MedPAC understood that the rarity of adverse events in home health care makes adverse events more difficult to risk adjust, which has been the main flaw in OBQM measures. Nonetheless, adding risk-adjusted adverse event measures to pay for performance could help to enhance patient safety. MedPAC also suggested that measures of processes related to patient safety would need to be developed. Unless there is a major shift in politics, home health care is likely to see pay for performance in late 2009 or 2010.

PROCESS MEASURES

High-quality health care is clinically appropriate and evidence-based. One of the current weaknesses of measuring quality in home health care is the lack of standardized tools to look at the process of care delivery. Individual organizations address this issue by developing their own measures, but the lack of uniformity limits comparison across agencies. There is debate going on currently within CMS about the possibility of requiring process measures at the patient level in the next revision of OASIS. "OASIS-C" might include measures related to whether the patient has received vaccinations (eg, influenza, pneumococcal), pain interventions, foot examinations, risk assessment for falls, and medication reconciliation. In addition to outcomes measure by OASIS-B, OASIS-C would allow agencies to assess whether process improvements lead to better outcomes. Mandating the measurement of process by CMS would create additional information that could be used to compare agencies and may become part of public reporting and eventually pay for performance. Undoubtedly, home health care agencies will be concerned about the increased burden of collecting the information, but the potential value to improve the quality of care could be substantial.

PATIENT SATISFACTION

Another major component in care quality is the patient's view of the care delivered. Measuring consumer satisfaction in home health care has occurred for years, with various vendors surveying patients (eg, Gallop, Press Ganey) and providing "benchmark" reports comparing data from agencies to national data. Most surveys require patients to rate on a scale (eg, 1 = poor to 5 = excellent) how satisfied they were with different aspects of the care delivered. As an example, Press Ganey asks about the admissions process, nurses, therapists, home health aides, and discharge process. Similar surveys have been used in hospitals for many years. As with hospitals, CMS has been pushing toward the use of a universal tool that would allow home health agencies to assess not only satisfaction with care but also the overall patient experience. Measures of this type have already been designed and tested for hospitals.[15] The measure used in hospitals is called the Consumer Assessment of Healthcare Providers and Systems (CAHPS).

The Agency for Healthcare Research and Quality is developing a measure for home health care to be called Home Health CAHPS. The new measure would focus on the patient's perspective on the care delivery process: did home health care start as soon as needed, did someone talk to you about your medications, did someone look at all your prescriptions, and did the care providers listen to your needs? The overall approach is to go beyond global impressions about the care and to rate more than satisfaction alone. As with other providers, CMS will eventually mandate CAHPS for home health care. Implementation could occur as early as 2010. HCAHPS will likely become part of public reporting and pay for performance.

QUALITY INITIATIVES IN HOME HEALTH CARE
Local Examples

The Plan, Do, Study, Act (PDSA) approach to quality improvement[16] has been adopted by many home health agencies. PDSA is based on the principle that small tests of change should be initiated before the organization makes a major commitment to formal changes in how care is delivered. For example, if patients complain in patient satisfaction surveys that nurses are not telling them about scheduled visits, the agency could test a new policy about prior notification in one geographic area and look for changes in satisfaction levels before agency-wide implementation. The PDSA approach has been used by home health agencies to improve the quality of OASIS information collected on patients. Stadt and Molare[17] found that agencies were able to improve the accuracy of OASIS documentation of the patients' condition at the start of care. Various "best practices" were identified that could be implemented at all home health care agencies: regular education about OASIS items, use of patient demonstration instead of interviewing, collaboration among disciplines in the completion of the assessment, clinical supervisors reviewing the documentation for completeness, and integration of OASIS into the comprehensive assessment.

Some quality improvement projects have focused on specific clinical issues. For example, PDSA methodology has been used in improving how nurses help patients manage pain.[18] At one agency, the efforts improved patient outcomes to exceed national benchmarks. Pain management became "an intrinsic patient care activity that reflects itself in language, demeanor and documentation of caregivers of this home care department."[18] The biggest application of PDSA and, by far, the most extensive efforts to improve home health care quality have been to reduce the number of acute care hospitalizations. The February 2008 issue of *Home Health Care Management & Practice* was devoted to quality improvement, and almost every article touched on reducing hospitalization rates, with many authors reporting positive results. The topics included risk assessment,[19] medication management[20] telehealth[21] and physician communication.[22] As can be seen in these articles, there is a serious agenda currently underway in home health care to improve the care delivered.

Balanced Scorecards

As home health agencies have grown more sophisticated in collecting data, there has been increasing reliance on balanced scorecards. The scorecards are used to report information to senior management and the board of trustees of the agency. These scorecards typically include measures of process, outcomes, use, satisfaction, human resources, and financial performance. The outcome measures rely on OBQI and OBQM measures derived from OASIS. Utilization data are captured on census, volume, length of stay, number of professional service visits (eg, nursing, physical therapy), and hours of paraprofessional services (eg, home health aides). Process measures represent the biggest challenge for agencies due to the lack of standardized measures and the need to collect data manually using medical record extraction. Examples include whether treatments follow the plan of care, wound care is appropriate, weights are taken for congestive heart failure patients, and foot exams are performed on diabetics. Satisfaction measures are based on surveys of patients and caregivers. Human resources measures focus on turnover rates, number of positions that need to be filled, recruitment rates, and overall "head count." The finance metrics include profit (for-profit agencies) or margin (not-for-profit agencies), days outstanding in accounts receivable, percentage of managed care patients, and average number of visits per Medicare PPS episode. Scorecards usually include several domains formatted to fit on one page.

The Visiting Nurse Service of New York (VNSNY) is one of the largest not-for-profit home health agencies and has been using a balanced scorecard for more than 5 years, which includes process, use, outcome, and satisfaction measures (**Fig. 1** presents an example). Each year, a new scorecard is developed depending on the performance on certain measures, high-priority agency initiatives, or areas targeted for improvement. VNSNY sets targets for every scorecard measure and assesses performance through the year. Scorecards are distributed throughout the agency and presented at board meetings.

Collaboratives Based on IHI Model

The Institute for Healthcare Improvement (IHI) developed an approach that combines the PDSA improvement methodology with systematic rollout of changes across an organization with multiple operational units or across health care industry groups called collaboratives. The idea is for individual units (eg, teams, agencies) to test changes, identify what works, and spread the improvements across the other sites. The process is predicated on the idea that there will be early and late adopters, but eventually all sites will benefit.

The ReACH (reducing acute care hospitalizations) National Demonstration Collaborative[23] is an example of how the IHI approach has been applied to home health care. ReACH is a 2-year multiwave initiative using the collaborative model to reduce acute care hospitalizations among home health care patients. Using a combination of virtual

Quality Score Card

Report Coverage: Jan 2007 to Dec 2007
Program Selected: A - Adult Acute Care
Region Selected: ALL - All Borough
Team Selected: ALL - All Team

Process Measures	Target	Monthly	Actual YTD	Outcomes Measures	Target	Monthly	Actual YTD
Care Management Documentation (**)	83.0%	79.8%	78.2%	All Dx: Overall Hospitalization Rate (**)	27.4%	24.8%	26.9%
Diabetic Care		82.5%	82.2%	% to hospitalization-OBQI episode 1-3 days		7.6%	8.2%
Wound Care		78.8%	75.9%	% to hospitalization-OBQI episode 4-60 days		76.5%	72.9%
CHF Care		72.5%	69.5%	% to hospitalization-OBQI episode 61-120 days		7.4%	9.0%
HHA Oversight (**)	80.0%	81.4%	80.0%	% to hospitalization-OBQI episode >120 days		8.5%	10.0%
Care Provided consistent with PPOC		89.6%	86.7%	All Dx: Overall Hospitalization Rate (Active Census)	9.5%	8.8%	9.8%
Supervision is documented every 14 days		81.3%	80.0%	Improvement in ADL's (OBQI) (**)			
Compliance with completion of HHA Task tool at SOC and Re-evaluation		79.0%	75.7%	Bathing	66.9%	65.4%	66.8%
Discharge Planning				Transferring	56.7%	50.6%	54.0%
Documentation of Discharge plan for patients by 120 days	85.0%	85.5%	82.6%	Ambulation	42.2%	41.7%	43.2%
				Management of Oral Medications	51.2%	52.8%	53.1%

Cost Measures	Target	Monthly	Actual YTD	Satisfaction Measures	Target	Monthly	Actual YTD
PPS visits per episode				Overall Satisfaction	83.0	83.2	83.0
Medicare	25.6	23.5	24.7	Communication with home care team (**)			
Professional		17.6	18.5	Dealing with the Office	80.0	77.6	77.5
RN		9.9	10.4				
Rehab		7.3	7.8				
SW		0.3	0.3				
Paraprofessional		6.0	6.2				
Dually Eligible	36.5	33.1	36.4				
Professional		17.3	18.3				
RN		11.9	12.7				
Rehab		5.2	5.3				
SW		0.2	0.3				
Paraprofessional		15.8	18.1				
HHA Utilization							
HHA Utilization matches assessed need	85.0%	95.0%	91.0%				

Fig. 1. Example of balanced scorecard. (*Courtesy of* Visiting Nurse Service of New York, New York, NY; with permission.)

and face-to-face communications, ReACH provided agencies access to improvement methods, training, and technical assistance. Agencies learned about risk assessment tools, recommendations for practice change, how to use standardized measures, and how to monitor hospitalization outcomes. Agencies were free to choose what was implemented at their organization. Boyce and Feldman[23] found that local improvement efforts were based on strategies disseminated by the collaborative: instituting care plans based on patient risk for hospitalization, front loading visits for high-risk patients, developing emergency response plans for patients, using disease management tools, and improving nursing/physician communication. Based on interviews with high-performing agencies, among those that had the greatest reduction of hospitalizations compared with baseline, there was a common consensus that the ReACH collaborative was a key component in their success.

CMS—8th Scope of Work

In 2005, CMS contracted with QIOs across the country to focus on reducing avoidable hospitalizations in home health care as part of the 8th Scope of Work (SOW). One goal of the 8th SOW was to reduce hospitalizations during home health care to 23% by August 2007. QIOs were instructed to identify tools and resources to assist home health care agencies with their improvement efforts. The Medicare Quality Improvement Community Web site (www.MedQIC.org) was developed to be the one-stop place for the quality improvement tools and resources.[24] Between August and December 2006, there were 120 tools and resources posted to the Web site, including diverse information on publicly reported hospitalization rates, organization culture, telehealth, and adult immunizations. QIOs worked more intensively with approximately 20% of the home health agencies across the country and less intensively with the remainder to reduce hospitalizations. After 1 year, agencies that worked more intensively with the QIOs reduced their hospitalization rates to 26%, while the others remained at 28%.[20] This is a similar impact as was seen in the initial large national OBQI demonstration in which agencies lowered adjusted hospitalization rates from 33% to 29% and then to 25% in a 3-year period.[21] Clearly, there is additional room for improvement, and a 2008 study showed that early adopters were able to achieve a relative 5% improvement in hospitalization rate.[22]

Accreditation: Joint Commission and Community Health Accreditation Program

In many areas of health care, accreditation bodies have traditionally driven quality improvement. This is less true for home health care than for other sectors, particularly hospitals. The Joint Commission and the Community Health Accreditation Program (CHAP), respectively, accredit similar numbers of home health agencies. The trend is for hospital-based agencies to seek Joint Commission accreditation, whereas freestanding agencies prefer CHAP. These accrediting bodies have had limited influence in the past because their standards were less focused on specific issues that could affect direct care delivery. However, both the Joint Commission and CHAP are changing their requirements in ways that will more directly influence home health care quality.

For example, the 2008 National Patient Safety Goals[23] have great potential to make agencies more accountable for "hand off" communications, medication administration, medication reconciliation, reducing infections, falls prevention, encouraging patient and family involvement in safety, using patient risk assessments to avoid adverse events, and conducting home safety risk assessments (eg, working smoke detectors).

CHAP's mandate is that each agency has a performance improvement process that integrates the organization's mission and ties it to patient outcomes.[24] There is an emphasis on measuring outcomes, benchmarking, evaluating progress in meeting improvement goals, measuring patient satisfaction, and ensuring that quality information is reported to the governing board. There is much latitude in how each agency meets the standards. Nonetheless, the focus on outcomes and the evaluation process pushes agencies in a direction that should improve care delivery.

National Quality Forum

In 2005, the National Quality Forum (NQF) released a report on its efforts to develop consensus standards for home health care.[25] The report included a framework for measuring home health care services, which focused on outcomes, process, and structure. The framework for these domains is presented in **Table 3**. NQF recommended that 6 priority areas should determine the guiding principles of measurement. First, measures are in regular, widespread use and/or required for other purposes. Second, some of the measures must apply to all home health care patients. Third, some of the measures must apply to all home health care organizations. Fourth, measures address high-risk, high-volume, and/or high-cost conditions or treatments. Fifth, measures address the six NQF focus domains: safe, beneficial, patient-centered, timely, efficient, and equitable. Sixth, measures address priorities for national health care quality recommended by the Institute of Medicine. In addition, NQF proposed that 15 evidence-based performance measures be collected to compare agencies

Table 3
National Quality Forum recommendations for outcome, process, and structure measures
Outcomes (quality of life and quality of care)
Utilization outcomes
Functional
Physiological
Cognitive
Emotional/behavioral
Perception of care
Safety
Process
Referral/intake
Patient assessment
Care planning and implementation of treatment
Education and consultation to patient and family
Care coordination and continuity
Participation in care management (patient and caregiver)
Structure
Results of external assessments
System and organization characteristics including use, costs, etc
Workforce and human resources characteristics

and made recommendations for implementation. The measures parallel those available via OBQI and are included in **Table 4**.

Perhaps one of the most important issues for the advancement of quality improvement in home health care is the identification of priority areas of research that would lead to the development of new measures. Four criteria were proposed for evaluation and selection of measures: importance, scientific acceptability, usability, and feasibility. Examples of these new measures can be found in **Table 5**. Clearly, if these measures were adopted, the assessment of quality would become more robust and comprehensive.

THE NEAR FUTURE

The specifics of the next phase of quality improvement for the Medicare QIO program, the 9th SOW, are expected in late 2008 but are not yet public. However, some themes are clear and represent a convergence of Medicare initiatives and efforts by the NQF, the Joint Commission, the IHI, and other groups and organizations that are engaged in pushing the national quality agenda.

Patient safety will likely be a central theme, including avoidance of medication errors and preventable complications, such as pressure ulcers and intravenous line infections. Related to this theme will be provider credentialing, with the underlying expectation that those delivering care are qualified for their work. Medicare has a legal mandate to ensure, to the extent possible, that beneficiaries are protected from harm resulting from the actions of health care providers and the health care system in general. Current discussions of pay for performance and other ways of differentially compensating providers based on the quality of care connect directly to the theme of accountability and safety.

Table 4
Outcome measures recommended by National Quality Forum

15 Standardized performance measures to compare home health care providers
Improvement in ambulation/locomotion
Improvement in bathing
Improvement in transferring
Improvement in management of oral medications
Improvement in pain interfering with activity
Improvement in status of surgical wounds
Improvement in dyspnea
Improvement in urinary incontinence
Increase in number of pressure ulcers
EC for wound infections, deteriorating wound status
EC for improper medication administration, medication side effects
EC for hypo/hyperglycemia
Acute care hospitalization
Discharge to community
Emergent care

Going forward, we can anticipate increasing focus on extended episodes of care across settings or even longitudinal care of selected individuals, rather than setting-specific outcomes. This would incorporate care transitions, which are appropriately selected for attention though not yet sufficiently well addressed in measurement and enforcement. The patient assessment and care process measures to

Table 5
National Quality Forum research priorities for new measures

Suggested new measures
Adequacy of support services post-discharge
Standardized pain scales
Refinement of measuring wound healing
Depression
Cognitive impairment
Quality of life
Patient perception of functional status
Physiological measures
Risk assessment and associated interventions (eg, falls)
Behavior change and compliance
Choice of home health care provider
Chronic illness support, disease management
Vaccinations
Discharge appropriateness
Unmet patient needs
Efficiency, cost savings of home health care
Patient and family satisfaction with services and providers

support this agenda are still being improved and developed. OASIS, the mainstay of home care quality measurement, will soon be re-issued as OASIS-C. The continuity assessment record and evaluation (CARE) instrument, which is intended to cross settings, is in pilot tests. Moving from the current scenario, which has a collection of setting-specific measures (OASIS for home care, minimum data set [MDS] for nursing homes), will be costly because these measures are deeply imbedded in extensive operational systems and require research to show that new measures are valid for measuring risk-adjusted outcomes, which will probably affect provider income.

Those involved in home care may view this scenario with mixed feelings. The general interest in advanced chronic illness care, care coordination, and care transitions is encouraging. There is a risk that providers who care for the sickest patients may be disadvantaged by using quality measures developed in other areas of health care, which are often based on data from younger populations and patients with individual conditions rather than those with extensive comorbidity. To date, most selected quality measures have not incorporated multimorbidity, and many are setting-specific. Consider the most widely cited quality measures, such as the A1c hemoglobin and other process measures related to diabetic care or prescription of beta blockers for patients with acute coronary artery disease in the hospital; these highlight the focus on the disease rather than on the whole patient. The measures recommended by a workgroup that reviewed the Assessing Care of Vulnerable Elders guidelines suggest a better approach to the care of chronically ill homebound patients.[26] These measures place a greater emphasis on quality of life and may hold the key to future measures of home care quality.

REFERENCES

1. Shaughnessy PW, Crisler KS. Outcome-based quality improvement: a manual for home care agencies on how to use outcomes. Washington, DC: National Association of Home Care; 1995.
2. Shaughnessy PW, Crisler KS, Schlenker RE, et al. Measuring and assuring the quality of home health care. Health Care Financ Rev 1994;16(1):35–67.
3. Shaughnessy P, Crisler K, Schlenker R. Medicare's OASIS: standardized outcome and assessment information set for home health care: OASIS-B. Denver (CO): Center for Health Services and Policy Research; 2002.
4. Hittle DF, Shaughnessy PW, Crisler KS, et al. A study of reliability and burden of home health assessment using OASIS. Home Health Care Serv Q 2003;22(4): 43–63.
5. Madigan EA, Fortinsky RH. Interrater reliability of the outcomes and assessment information set: results from the field. Gerontologist 2004;44(5):689–92.
6. Neder S, Rosati RJ, Huang L. Assessment of OASIS inter-rater reliability and validity using several methodological approaches. Home Health Care Serv Q 2005; 24(3):23–38.
7. Shaughnessy P, Crisler K, Schlenker R, et al. OASIS. The next 10 years. Caring 1998;17(6):32–4, 36, 38.
8. Egger E. Jefferson home care sees OASIS not as a burden, but a tool to improve performance. Health Care Strateg Manage 1999;17(5):14–5.
9. Conway KS, Richard AA. Unexpected benefits of OASIS and OBQI. Home Healthc Nurse 2000;18(4):255–7.
10. Shaughnessy P, Hittle D. Overview of risk adjustment and outcome measures for home health agency OBQI reports: highlights of current approaches and outline

of planned enhancements. Denver (CO): Center for Health Services and Policy Research; 2002.

11. Department of Health and Human Services. Medicare program: prospective payment system for home health agencies. Fed Regist 2000;65(128):41128–214.

12. Department of Health and Human Services. Medicare program: prospective payment system refinement and rate update for calendar year 2008. Fed Regist 2007;72(86):25356–481.

13. Centers for Medicare and Medicaid Services. Appendix: guidelines for reviewing case mix and adverse event outcome reports. Available at: http://www.cms.hhs.gov/HomeHealthQualityInits/Downloads/HHQIOASISOBQMAppendix.pdf; 2001. Accessed July 31, 2008.

14. Pay for Performance: Committee on Finance, US Senate, July 25, 2005 (Testimony of Mark E. Miller, Executive Director, Medicare Payment Advisory Commission).

15. CAHPS® hospital survey chartbook: what patients say about their experiences with hospital care. AHRQ Publication No. 07-0064-EF. Rockville (MD): Agency for Healthcare Research and Quality; May 2007.

16. Deming WE. Massachusetts institute of technology center for advanced engineering study. Cambridge (MA): Out of Crisis; 1992.

17. Stadt J, Molare E. Best practices: that improved patient outcomes and agency operational performance. Home Healthc Nurse 2005;23(9):587–93.

18. Goodman D, Hiniker PB, Paley JM. How to improve home care pain management processes. Home Healthc Nurse 2003;21(5):325–34.

19. Anderson D, Backaler M. Hospitalization and emergent care risk assessment. Home Health Care Management & Practice 2008;20(2):117–24.

20. Chetney R. Using telehealth to avoid urgent care and hospitalization. Home Health Care Management & Practice 2008;20(2):117–24.

21. Markley J, Winbery S. Communicating with physicians: How agencies can be heard. Home Health Care Management & Practice 2008;20(2):161–8.

22. McDonald MV, Peterson LE. Finding success in medication management. Home Health Care Management & Practice 2008;20(2):135-40.

23. Boyce PS, Feldman PH. ReACH National demonstration collaborative: early results of implementation. Home Health Care Serv Q 2007;27(4):105–20.

24. Essay M. The QIO program, home health and the national acute care hospitalization priority. Home Health Care Management & Practice 2008;20(2):110–6.

25. Shaughnessy PW, Hittle DF, Crisler KS, et al. Improving patient outcomes of home health care: findings from two demonstration trials of outcome-based quality improvement. J Am Geriatr Soc 2002;50(8):1354–64.

26. Medicare Quality Improvement Organization Support Center for Home Health (2008). Final Evaluation Report June 2008, Report prepared by Quality Insights of Pennsylvania, Under contract with Centers for Medicare and Medicaid Services, Publication Number 8SOW-PA-HHQ08.8002.

Care Transitions and Home Health Care

Peter A. Boling, MD

KEYWORDS

- Transitional care • Transitions of care • Home care
- Home health care • Discharge planning

Care transitions are finally receiving much-needed attention by health services researchers and quality of care advocates, but the problems are serious, and we are far from an acceptable level of performance.[1] Transitions of care are defined as "a set of actions designed to ensure the coordination and continuity of health care as patients transfer between different locations or different levels of care in the same location."[2] Although transition problems have long been familiar and troubling to busy clinicians, progress in quality improvement has been hindered by measurement and attribution challenges and lack of focused attention by those making health policy. Furthermore, even now when transition problems are better recognized, neither health care providers nor those directing health care quality and payment policy have systematically and adequately addressed them. Despite increasing awareness of the problem, and explicit policies by government and other quality advocates that have existed for many years, care is still delivered by organizations that effectively operate in silos, and most handoffs are unacceptably poor, creating a serious quality problem and substantial danger for patients.

A typical example of in-home care is a hospital discharge with follow-up care by a home health agency and primary care physician. The post-acute care providers are not involved during the hospitalization and receive little or no direct communication from the hospital on discharge. Although thoughtful, documented inpatient discharge planning efforts are normative, including attempted medication reconciliation, this work is usually lost in transition. Medication reconciliation in the hospital is often flawed because of inaccurate baseline data, involving hurried physicians who are often rotating and using increasingly complex and mutually exclusive data systems, and in some cases by lack of attention to detail. Transfer documents are often inadequate: they are brief, handwritten, and illegible; they address only portions of the care plan; they lack most of the important clinical details from the hospital course and inpatient care plan; and too often, they contain errors.

The home health agency constructs a care plan anew using limited documents that went home with the patient together with information obtained during the in-home

Department of Medicine, Virginia Commonwealth University, PO Box 980102, Richmond, VA 23298, USA
E-mail address: pboling@mcvh-vcu.edu

Clin Geriatr Med 25 (2009) 135–148
doi:10.1016/j.cger.2008.11.005
0749-0690/08/$ – see front matter © 2009 Elsevier Inc. All rights reserved.

geriatric.theclinics.com

assessment from patient and family. In the home are multiple medication bottles of varied ages bearing several physicians' names from before the hospitalization and new discharge medications with new physician names, often with no refills. There may be redundancy, therapeutic duplication, and dose discrepancies. Some pre-scribed medications are absent because of miscommunication, noncompliance, lack of finances, or formulary mismatches. If the agency staff requests more informa-tion from the hospital, they may be told, although incorrectly, that the Health Insurance Portability and Accountability Act precludes sharing information without additional written permission. If they attempt to call a hospital-based provider who knows the case, they are likely to be seeking someone who is difficult to identify or unavailable, and knowing this, they may not try.

Weeks later, an office-based primary care physician receives home care orders to sign, which may be the first time that the physician knows of the hospital admission. The wealth of information obtained during the intensive, costly inpatient stay is largely inaccessible to longitudinal medical care providers outside the hospital system. Usu-ally, these providers in turn are remotely and passively involved in the immediate post-hospital care, which is managed almost entirely by the home health agency.

The flaws in this prevalent scenario probably contribute to the 28% average read-mission rate of Medicare home health care patients during the first 60 days of home care, which is a publicly reported, high-profile quality indicator.

This article summarizes the literature on hazards of care transitions and evidence for models designed to improve care during transitions. The focus is on transitions into home health care, but the same principles apply when home health patients are sent to a hospital or nursing home or when home health patients are discharged to independent self-care.

PREVALENCE AND TYPOLOGY OF TRANSITION PROBLEMS

Experts have drawn attention to the high frequency of patients returning to hospitals shortly after entering post-acute care. Kane[3] reported the following rates of rehospi-talization within 30 days after discharge for selected common diagnoses (**Table 1**).

Several authors have further categorized and quantified transition problems. Earlier work by Murtaugh used 1994 National Long-Term Care Survey data and found that in a 2-year period there were 15 million transitions in the 5-million-person sample frame.[4] Of these persons, 18% had a post-acute or long-term care transitional event, and 9% had seven or more transitions. Most concerning was that 1.1 million persons or 22% of those with transitions had administrative data pointing to possible system failures: in-tercurrent emergency room (ER) visits or potentially avoidable hospitalizations.

Table 1 Post-hospital readmission rates		
Diagnosis (Initial)	30-day Readmission (%)	60-day Readmission (%)
Hip fracture	12.14	18.38
Pneumonia	16.18	21.12
Stroke	15.51	22.76
COPD	18.35	21.12
Congestive heart failure	23.30	33.95

Abbreviation: COPD, chronic obstructive pulmonary disease.

Coleman and colleagues more recently analyzed the Medicare Current Beneficiary Survey looking at a 30-day period following hospital discharge and found 46 service use patterns. Of the initial post-hospital transfers, 74% went home and 16% involved a rehabilitation facility, including nursing homes. Most patients (61%) had a single transfer, but many had two (18%), three (8%), and more (4%); the remainder died during the 30-day period.[5] Another analysis by Coleman and others compared managed care and fee-for-service patients, finding that one in seven patients discharged from hospitals had four to six transitions within 3 months.[6] As a primary care provider who seeks to follow such people longitudinally, the author finds that they are often tumbling through the health care system.

Wolff and colleagues[7] have just reported that most patients admitted to Medicare Part A home health care in 2004 came from other institutional care settings: hospitals (50%), nursing facilities (18%), or inpatient rehabilitation facilities (8%). Subsequently, more than one-third of patients discharged from home care received institutional care in hospitals (29%) and nursing facilities (8%) within 30 days.

Stroke patients are often rehospitalized (20%). Kind studied data on stroke patients from 11 metropolitan regions who were discharged to post-acute care settings in 1998–2000 following an ischemic stroke and were readmitted within 30 days. The patients, who averaged slightly more than 80 years of age, were in Medicare managed care plans (570 stroke patients) and fee-for-service Medicare (4,680 stroke patients).[8] Of 5,250 patients, 3,683 had one readmission and survived, 671 died during a bounce-back admission, and 896 had multiple return admissions. Aspiration pneumonia was the most common readmission diagnosis, and heart disease was second.

The problems that occur during transitions from one care setting to the next have also been codified, and the predominant categories are no surprise; medication management and continuity of the care plan lead the list. Medication management is a key component as reviewed by Foust and coworkers.[9] Based on chart reviews, and acknowledging that limitation, Moore and colleagues found that 49% of patients discharged from hospital with clinic follow-up had lapses related to medications, test follow-up, or completion of a planned workup; medication discrepancies (42%) were the most prevalent.[10] Boockvar and coworkers determined that in transfers between four hospitals and two nursing homes, three medications were changed on average, and 20% of patients had a resulting adverse drug event.[11] Forster and colleagues found that 19% of patients discharged from hospitals had one or more adverse events within 3 weeks; a third were considered preventable, and adverse drug events were the most common of these (66%).[12] Coleman and coauthors found that 14% of post-hospital transitions to home included medication discrepancies[13] and have stated that shortfalls in handoff documents are "too numerous to count." Wong and colleagues studied post-hospital care, finding unintentional medication discrepancies in 41%, with incomplete prescriptions and omitted medications being the most common; 29% of instances had the potential to affect outcomes.[14]

For many reasons, providers working in the hospital may find it difficult to determine reliably what medications the patient was taking before admission. Cornish and coworkers reported that 46% of hospitalized patients had one or more usual prescription medication(s) omitted without explanation; 39% risked potential harm.[15] An evidence review by the same group found 22 studies reporting that about two-thirds of hospitalized patients had incorrect histories regarding usual medications.[16] Common sense dictates that using an erroneous initial list makes discrepancies following discharge highly likely. Commitment, focused effort, and attention to detail are all required if this process is to be completed accurately. Often several phone calls are needed, to family caregivers, to primary care physicians, to pharmacies, and to home health agencies, to be confident of the result. Legible written instructions should be given to patients and caregivers, once the providers are clear about what the instructions should say.

INTERVENTIONS

There have been many studies of interventions designed to improve this generally dismal transitional care track record, and discharge planning and care coordination are not new ideas. In a 2008 Cochrane review, Mistaien and Poot found that simple telephonic interventions have not had consistent success despite a large number of studies.[17] Chiu and Newcomer also published an evidence review with 15 clinical trials conducted between 1999 and 2006, noting a variety of interventions, and reported that about half of the trials found reduced hospitalization in the intervention group.[18] Some examples of well-designed studies are discussed herein, and interventions are divided into two groups based on intensity: the "coach," "guide," or system refinement approach and the "guardian angel" approach, which involves intensive case management by medical care providers.

Lower-Intensity Transition Interventions

After describing transition problems, Coleman and colleagues proposed a lower-intensity intervention that relies on four pillars: medication self-management; a patient-centered health record; arranged physician follow-up; and patient education regarding red flags, warning signs, and symptoms and how best to respond when these occur.[19] A randomized controlled study was conducted with about 375 patients per group in which experimental patients received information, coaching by an advance practice nurse, a home visit, and at least three telephone calls.[20] The 30-day hospitalization rate improved for the intervention patients (8.9%) compared with patients given usual care (13.8%). At 90 days, the difference was 13.5% compared with 22.9%. Mean hospital costs, using data from one large integrated delivery system, were $488 lower at 6 months. A national study of this approach is underway.

Boult and colleagues[21] at Johns Hopkins University are testing "guided care," which follows seven precepts of chronic care innovation (disease management, self-management, lifestyle modification, transitional care, caregiver education and support, health enhancement, and geriatric evaluation and management). A nurse, trained in this model and using evidence-based practices, carries a caseload of 50 to 60 patients served by a small number of primary care physicians (two to five). This study is in its early stages.

Simino and Feldman are using a collaborative approach to systematic quality improvement, working with a large number of home health agencies in a regional program called ReACH, which is aimed specifically at reducing acute care hospitalization.[22] Participating agencies take a standardized approach to identifying high-risk patients and share best practices to achieve improved outcomes. Initial results reflect the complexity of this task and the need to work hard to integrate care across settings.

Some lower-intensity models focus on a single health condition ("disease management"). These should be distinguished from models that address a wider range of comorbidities. One early and often cited report from Seattle involved hospitalized high-risk heart failure patients[23] who had multiple hospital admissions and heart failure related to ischemia or poorly controlled hypertension. In this randomized controlled trial, subjects received inpatient medication review by a geriatric cardiologist and specialized patient education combined with brief home care follow-up by a home health agency and telephonic contact with hospital-based staff. Readmissions dropped by half. This low-cost intervention has common features with the approach successfully tested by Coleman: continuity of the care plan, education of patient and caregiver, and extra attention paid at the point of greatest risk, the transition itself.

In general, disease management programs are designed to include large numbers of patients with a given single chronic disease, are not selective about enrollment criteria, are not well integrated with usual sources of medical care, and are not effective in lowering costs. Moreover, importantly, although certain diseases such as congestive heart failure unquestionably contribute to the rehospitalization problem, home health care is notably dominated by extensive comorbidity. For example, only 10% of hospitalizations during home care episodes are primarily caused by heart failure. Thus, disease-specific models may help in some patient subsets but will not solve most transition problems. Despite enormous resource investment, and some potential to delay onset of disease complications in healthier populations, disease management companies have generally not demonstrated value in the management of advanced chronic illness care (see the article by DeJonge, elsewhere in this issue).

Higher-Intensity Interventions

Naylor and colleagues[24] have experimented with a hospital-based approach to in-home intensive short-term medical case management. After an initial trial showed no difference in the early 1990s, a second was devised with a more intensive, longer intervention (4 weeks rather than 2 weeks) and an increasingly experienced staff. In this second randomized controlled trial, hospital-based advance practice nurses identified a high-risk group of inpatients, assessed them in the hospital, and followed them for a month, providing telephone support including evening and weekend hours plus multiple home visits (minimum of two, average of 4.5 visits), starting immediately after discharge. Rehospitalization and total health care costs were reduced by half, saving $3,031 per patient within 6 months after initial discharge.

Naylor's subjects were old (mean age, 75) and had a variety of primary diagnoses and an average of five active comorbidities, with other risk factors for turbulent post-hospital care. This study and others like it show that models targeting at-risk populations with a wide range of diagnoses and comorbidities can achieve a large, favorable impact. Naylor and colleagues have also applied intensive transitional care management to patients with congestive heart failure in another randomized controlled trial that found reduced readmissions (106 versus 162) after 1 year and lower costs ($4,845 lower per patient).[25]

Using a model of care designed like Naylor's and implemented starting in calendar year 2000, nurse practitioners at Virginia Commonwealth University (VCU) in Richmond, Virginia have managed more than 350 complex patients with a long list of diagnoses in an intensive short-term transitional care program.[26] Nearly three-quarters of the patients returned to office-based care, and 12% were transferred into the long-term house calls program for primary care when it became clear that return to office-based care was not possible. Health care costs measured by use of resources at VCU health system by the same patients for 6 months before and after transitional care were lower by 65% after enrollment.

Although not specifically a transitional care model, Phillips and colleagues[27] described a focused, closely managed longitudinal approach to the care of moderate-risk elders by a specialized office-based geriatric care team that developed within a later-stage social health maintenance organization (SHMO). Compared to usual multispecialty care, they found annual savings of $760 per patient in 2002. A subsequent adaptation called "office without walls" (OWW), their newest model, relies on home visits for medical care delivery and serves very frail patients with an average age of 87 years and 5.7 active medical problems. Analysis of data from 436 OWW patients compared with similar HMO patients in usual care indicates more than 50% reduction in hospitalization and savings of an estimated $1.5 million per year when adjusted to a 1,000-patient reference standard (Phillips SL, personal communication of unpublished data. May 2007).[28]

COMPARING AND CONTRASTING MODELS

Despite the heterogeneous mixture of negative and positive studies in the discharge planning literature, it is clear that a carefully designed, appropriately targeted intervention performed by a well-prepared team is able to achieve impressive reductions in hospital admissions and total costs of care. This brings to mind similar observations made about outcomes of surgery, patient selection, and provider experience. It is also likely that there are mitigating factors and that several different models can be effective.

One of the mitigating factors is local practice environment. During the early years of Medicare managed care, the large profits generated by HMOs that operated in very high-cost geographic regions highlighted the opportunity to reduce costs in communities where there is much discretionary care. Recent reports on the care of patients with advanced chronic illness in the last 2 years of life from Wennberg and colleagues' group at Dartmouth show that there is still marked regional variation in health care expenditures, including hospitalization.[28] State-to-state these differences are twofold or more, and higher spending is not connected to better outcomes.[28] Local supply of hospital beds and specialists is one important driver of these practice pattern differences. In turn, local practices engender expectations by patients and establish community standards that medical practitioners consider when choosing management strategies for acute illness. Marked variations in use like this indicate an opportunity to improve care systems while lowering costs.

Here it is worth mentioning again the author's decades of experience in Richmond, Virginia, where there is very little Medicare risk contracting and where there are three large competing health systems (academic, for-profit, and not-for-profit) that all have electronic clinical data systems. Virginia's statewide health care costs are relatively low as are average adjusted per capita costs in the Richmond region. Yet, in this community, the care of patients with advanced chronic illness remains fragmented, discontinuous, and fraught with peril as they move from one setting to the next. Notably, the intensive care management teams at the author's institution have markedly improved these care patterns, suggesting that even in lower-cost regions there are opportunities to improve care and lower costs.

One exception to the common rule of fragmented care may lie in some integrated health systems.[29] Here again, the literature is limited and inconsistent. There are accounts of low-intensity care coordination programs that failed to improve the bottom line within managed care organizations.[30] There have also been failures reported in nurse-led HMO programs focused on diseases such as heart failure that have been selected for proactive management.[31] However, other reports from managed care organizations suggest that 50% savings are achievable.[32]

Another important influence is the way that the new model is implemented, including the characteristics of the providers involved. A case in point is the national home-based primary care trial conducted within the Veterans Affairs (VA) system a decade ago, using 16 sites. Attempts were made to standardize care processes, yet although 15 of 16 sites targeted high-risk patients, only 9 (56%) involved the home based primary care (HBPC) team in discharge planning, and only 11 (68%) provided 24-hour phone support to patients.[33] Effective intervention during intervals of high medical instability requires clinical experience, comfort and skill with complex decisions, detailed knowledge of the patient, prompt availability when needed, and relationships with other key health care resources that are needed to successfully resolve the instability.

One of the important questions to be answered about the solutions to the transition problem is the extent to which empowered patients and family caregivers can assume responsibility for coordinating care. There is evidence that when patients and families are given useful tools and coached, rehospitalization is reduced, satisfaction is improved, and money can be saved. This in turn depends on the financial resources, innate coping skills, and educational attainment of the patient and family.

However, some situations are simply too difficult for even the most adept patient or lay caregivers to handle with a brief coaching assistance during the initial transition. The coaching approach is prone to failure when the medical care plan requires early and frequent revision or when caregivers and patients themselves are not able to deal with the complexity of the health problems and health system hurdles. Particular examples include patients with multiple unstable interacting health conditions or dependence on advanced medical technology and families with limited economic resources or low health literacy. Even highly educated and affluent individuals are sometimes challenged by today's sophisticated medical therapies and the health system's incongruities.

With these caveats and making a very rough estimate of relative value, one can perceive a possible dose–response gradient when cost savings are considered in relation to intensity from recent randomized controlled trials of transitional care interventions, as shown in **Table 2**.

Such comparisons must be made cautiously. Hospital costs for usual care patients were far higher in Naylor's study from the late 1990s ($5,500 per person) than the usual care patients' hospital costs in Coleman's 2002 clinical trial ($2,500 per person). The hospitals in Naylor's 1999 report are large eastern urban university medical centers with their attendant complexities, whereas Coleman studied patients in a western integrated health system. The author's experience at VCU medical center appears more similar to that in Naylor's 1999 report.

KEY PERSONNEL NEEDED FOR IMPROVED CARE TRANSITIONS

Other considerations include ease of implementing interventions and availability of staff with necessary skills. Many of the models described above have employed nurse

Table 2
Three randomized controlled trials of transitional care teams

Author	Setting	Clinical Focus	Subjects per Group	Years	Duration	Intensity	Savings/ Patient ($)
Naylor et al	2 university hospitals	Varied	180	1992–1996	6 months	High	$3,301
Naylor et al	6 urban hospitals	Heart failure	120	1997–2001	12 months	High	$4,845
Coleman et al	HMO, 1 hospital, 8 NHs, 1 HHA	Varied	370	2002–2003	6 months	Low	$488

Abbreviations: HHA, home health agency; NHs, nursing homes.

practitioners and other advance practice nurses, linked to varying degrees with physicians who are often hospital-based to support the medical decision making. Such interdisciplinary teams constitute a well-established strategy in geriatric care. Transitional care requires an experienced and committed staff that is comfortable with independent work roles and very sick patients. It is advantageous to be based at the hospital since this is where the team initially finds the patients, the clinical records, and the inpatient providers to build the front end of the bridge. Team chemistry, focus, and relationships with other providers at the hospital affect the outcomes and team durability. It took more than a year to develop the current successful model at VCU medical center, starting with an experienced group of nurse practitioners and an established house calls program for a base of operations.

Only a fraction of hospital inpatients need the extra help offered by specialized transitional care teams. Experience in case finding and having defined criteria help the teams to identify the patients who will most likely benefit from intensive transitional care efforts. Staff development, regular meetings, and recognition of the team's value are important. Intensive models serve small numbers of patients. Program evaluation cannot be based on visit volumes but must focus on inpatient length of stay, readmission rates, and costs. In addition, with time it has been found that certain patients can be especially challenging, such as those with traumatic brain or spinal cord injury, ventilator dependence, polytrauma, and intravenous hyperalimentation.

An emerging phenomenon is the role of hospitalists who are physicians practicing exclusively in the hospital setting, providing acute care on a rotating, scheduled basis. Hospitalists are now an integral component of many health care systems, and these physicians are often involved in discharge planning for large proportions of a hospital's inpatients. Management of care transitions has not been routinely taught in the training of hospitalists, many of whom are recent graduates of internal medicine residency programs. Most hospitalists also have little familiarity with home health care or nursing home care. However, care transitions are becoming a defined element in the professional competencies for hospitalists,[34] and though this educational work is early in its development, it should improve the quality of transitions, especially as the infrastructure improves.

Traditional hospital discharge planners, who are usually nurses and social workers, should also have a specific performance improvement agenda. One facet is staff education. In particular, staff members who are hospital-based and have worked primarily in the hospital for extended periods often have limited, secondhand knowledge of external care environments: what external care providers can manage; what factors affect their decisions; and what they need from the hospital. Ongoing training that crosses sites of care would be worthwhile.

TRANSITIONS FROM NURSING HOME TO HOME CARE

The same considerations that apply to transitions from hospitals to home care also apply when patients leave the nursing home. A facility-based physician in the nursing home is commonly the attending physician of record there but usually is not the subsequent continuing care physician. The nursing home may have a formulary of its own, resulting again in medication regimen changes, and continuity of the care plan is rarely achieved. The outpatient physician who will follow the patient after discharge almost never receives direct contact or information from the nursing home around the time of discharge, and information sent to the home health agency is also typically limited. Since the transition home from the nursing home is one step removed from the earlier transfer from the hospital, whatever limited data the nursing home previously received from the hospital usually do not accompany the patient. In one study of medication reconciliation in the home following nursing home discharge in 521 HMO patients, Delate and coworkers disturbingly found that 73% had an inadvertent change in dosage, 48% had some drug omitted, and 19% had a therapeutic duplication.[35] Though the intervention did not affect ER use, the researchers reported fewer deaths among intervention patients.

TRANSITIONS FROM HOME TO HOSPITAL

Thus far, the discussion has focused on care transitions into home care from other care settings. The handoff of home care patients to hospitals or nursing homes also bears comment. Many of these transitions occur without the direct involvement or even knowledge of the home care provider, when the patient or family calls "911." However, in other cases, there is an opportunity for home care providers to inform the hospital in the same way that hospital providers should communicate with home health. This is rarely done and depends uniquely on the dedication and personal practices of the agency nurse rather than on standard agency procedures. Hospital ER providers complain as loudly about home care or nursing home patients who arrive with limited data as do post-acute care providers who experience this after hospital discharge. Whenever possible, providers at both ends of each handoff need to take ownership of the process.

INFORMATION TECHNOLOGY

The vision of a standard dataset or even an electronic health record that reliably follows patients across settings is often raised as a solution to transition problems. One can easily see how this could help. However, this solution is certainly years and probably decades away, will cost hundreds of billions of dollars to establish nationally, and will engender much acrimonious debate about which data systems will be used, who will control the data, which people will be allowed to access and edit the data, how data quality will be monitored, and where the data will reside. Anyone who has worked within a large health system as it implements an electronic health record will attest to those difficulties. Imagine then dealing with the complexities of working across numerous health systems and care silos: the proprietary business interests and the need to bridge mismatched formats and incompatible software systems will be a major challenge. Once these substantial hurdles are overcome, many of the current quality problems in care transitions may abate.

QUALITY IMPROVEMENT IN TRANSITIONAL CARE

Effective systematic quality improvement initiatives follow a defined process, such as "Plan, Do, Study, Act." The first steps are to define the problem and the measures of success. For transitions, Coleman and colleagues have proposed and validated one tool, the Care Transition Measure (CTM), which has been refined from a 15-item measure to a three item measure that is similarly valid[36,37] and reliably detects improved outcomes such as reduction in ER visits. The CTM depends on patient self-report, and the three-item version centers on how well the post-hospital care plan included patient preferences, patient education about health care, and information about medications. Since the CTM is based on self-report, it may work less well for populations who are less able to participate, and it does not capture the receiving provider perspective, which is also important. That is, it does not directly measure the work often required by those on the receiving end of transitions to restore the continuity of the care process after a suboptimal handoff.

Ultimately, providers must be accountable for their performance in order for change to occur. Although both CMS and the Joint Commission have for years required adequate handoffs, performance in this area is not scrutinized, and these standards have never been effectively enforced. The Joint Commission and other organizations interested in quality rely on anonymous patient satisfaction surveys as one measure that is gaining in importance. In an analogous strategy, one could imagine requiring hospitals and other organizations to conduct similar surveys of post-acute care providers regarding the perceived quality of the handoffs after transitions. Given the prevalence of problems and the nearly universal frustration of post-acute providers with this aspect of health care, it is suspected that the initial results would be telling.

SCOPE OF THE CHALLENGE AND NECESSARY NEXT STEPS

A relatively small subset of people, mostly elderly, who are medically complex and frail, are likely to incur frequent major expenses associated with episodes of worsening health. Most of these people live in the community with high-grade functional impairment and extensive comorbidity. Based on demographic and health care use data, they number 2 to 3 million now but will probably reach 6 million by 2025. Researchers at the University of Michigan have also used administrative data to estimate the size of the population likely to benefit from intensive care management, similarly finding that about 2 million people would currently be eligible for care coordination if the criteria were more than 3 complex medical problems or a cognitive deficit plus 1 or more functional deficits.[38] Because it may be possible to reduce recurrent hospital admissions in members of this subpopulation by as much as 50% compared with usual care today, and because 10% of people use about 60% of health care resources, they should be the focus of intense interest.

Fig. 1 schematizes an approach to care for a community population. Within that population, the majority of people are basically healthy or are ambulatory with chronic

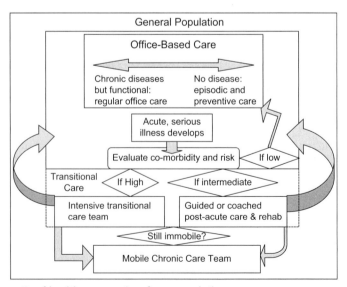

Fig. 1. Schematic of health care services for a population.

illnesses that need secondary prevention. Some of these people get acutely ill but rapidly recover. Assuming that they have health insurance, the majority of people are well served by office-based physicians. Other people develop more serious illnesses and ensuing functional deficits when they are acutely ill but recover after a period of variably intensive care management and rehabilitation (transitional care patients). A third group of people are so ill and functionally limited that they can never be managed effectively in an office-based care model and are best served by a mobile health care team for life.

To have safe and effective transitions in this or any model of care, providers must successfully complete a series of actions (**Table 3**) that have been frequently articulated in the context of discharge planning.

Medications deserve extra, focused attention, because errors are frequent and negative consequences are many. Recent changes in health care, particularly since the 2003 Medicare Modernization Act, have introduced new dimensions in the process. For example, many elderly outpatients now have prescription regimens that are painstakingly constructed to fit complex Medicare Part D coverage rules plus the patient's finances and prior health experiences, whereas hospitals have different formularies, and hospital-based physicians have their own preferred practices. It should be recognized that the brief hospital stay is a transient stop on the chronic care journey. There is little value in a neatly printed and legible list that is erroneous, inconsistent with the patient's insurance and thus unaffordable, or rife with unexplained and sometimes problematic discrepancies when compared with prior medications. Patients being returned to the community should be placed back on medications covered by their plans and medications prescribed by their longitudinal care providers unless there is a compelling clinical reason for changes.

Finally, the path through post-acute care, including nursing home care and home health care, is influenced by payer coverage and is likely to involve multiple transitions

Table 3	
Key elements in successful transitions	
Assessment of Need	**Medical, Functional, Cognitive and Behavioral, Support System**
Choose best next care setting	Nursing home Inpatient rehabilitation Assisted living Home with home health care Home with family or alone
Arrange services	Identify suitable agency(ies) and verify coverage
Patient and family education	Verbal Written (legible or printed)
Clinical summary	Course (diagnosis and treatment) Key data (laboratory, x-rays, other) Care plan's main elements (how to care for the patient)
Medication reconciliation	Current medication list What was stopped and why What was started and why
Follow-up medical care	Appointments (names, times, dates, phone numbers)

with multiple settings and multiple physicians. Therefore, the discharging team should think ahead and construct a care plan that brings the patient safely through an entire episode of illness with several stops along the way.

Transitions of care are hazardous times with much at stake. Following the airline industry analogy, brought prominently into the health policy dialog by the now famous Institute of Medicine report "To Err is Human," there should be a preflight checklist (see **Table 3**), and the flight should not leave the gate until all lights are green. When teaching about transitions, the author asks trainees to consider the needs of the patient, the family, and the providers that will assume responsibility for the medical care plan. "Put yourself in their shoes for a minute and then provide what you would want in their place" is sound advice and is the foundation of patient-centered care.

REFERENCES

1. Tsilimingras T, Bates DW. Addressing post-discharge adverse events: a neglected area. Jt Comm J Qual Patient Saf 2008;34(2):85–97.
2. Coleman EA, Berenson RA. Lost in transition: challenges and opportunities for improving the quality of transitional care. Ann Intern Med 2004;140:533–6.
3. Kane RL, Lin WC, Blewett LA. Geographic variation in the use of post-acute care. Health Serv Res 2002;37(3):667–82.
4. Murtaugh CM, Litke AL. Transitions through postacute and long-term care settings: patterns of use and outcomes for a national cohort of elders. Med Care 2002;40(3):227–36.
5. Coleman EA, Min SJ, Chomiak A, et al. Posthospital care transitions: patterns, complications and risk identification. Health Serv Res 2004;39(5):1449–65.
6. Ma E, Coleman EA, Fish R, et al. Quantifying posthospital care transitions in older patients. J Am Med Dir Assoc 2004;5(2):71–4.
7. Wolff JL, Meadow A, Weiss CO, et al. Medicare home health patients' transitions through acute and post-acute care settings. Med Care 2008;46(11):1188–93.
8. Kind AJH, Smith MA, Pandhi N, et al. Bouncing back: rehospitalization in patients with complicated transitions in the first thirty days after hospital discharge for acute stroke. Home Health Care Serv Q 2007;26(4):37–55.
9. Foust JB, Naylor MD, Boling PA, et al. Opportunities for improving post-hospital home medication management among older adults. Home Health Care Serv Q 2005;24(12):101–22.
10. Moore C, Wisnivesky J, Williams S, et al. Medical errors related to discontinuity of care from an inpatient to an outpatient setting. J Gen Intern Med 2003;18:646–51.
11. Boockvar K, Fishman E, Kyricacou CK, et al. Adverse events due to discontinuations in drug use and dose changes in patients transferred between acute and long-term care facilities. Arch Intern Med 2004;164:545–50.
12. Forster A, Murff H, Peterson J, et al. The incidence and severity of adverse events affecting patients after discharge from the hospital. Ann Intern Med 2003;138:161–7.
13. Coleman EA, Smith JD, Raha D, et al. Posthospital medication discrepancies: prevalence and contributing factors. Arch Intern Med 2005;165(16):1842–7.
14. Wong JD, Bajcar JM, Wong GG, et al. Medication reconciliation at hospital discharge. Ann Pharmacother 2008;42:1373–9.
15. Cornish PL, Knowles SR, Marchesano R, et al. Unintended medication discrepancies at the time of hospital admission. Arch Intern Med 2005;165:424–9.

16. Tam VC, Knowles SR, Cornish PL, et al. Frequency, type and clinical importance of medication history errors at admission to hospital: a systematic review. CMAJ 2005;173(5):510–5.

17. Mistaien P, Poot E. Telephone follow-up, initiated by a hospital-based health professional, for postdischarge problems in patients discharged from hospital to home (review). Cochrane Database Syst Rev 2006;(4):CD004510.

18. Chiu WK, Newcomer R. A systematic review of nurse-assisted case management to improve hospital discharge transition outcomes for the elderly. Prof Case Manag 2007;12(6):330–6.

19. Coleman EA, Smith JD, Frank JC, et al. Preparing patients and caregivers to participate in care delivered across settings: the care transitions intervention. J Am Geriatr Soc 2004;S2:1817–25.

20. Coleman EA, Parry C, Chalmers S, et al. The care transitions intervention: results of a randomized controlled trial. Arch Intern Med 2006;166:1822–8.

21. Boyd CM, Boult C, Shadmi E, et al. Guided care for multimorbid adults. Gerontologist 2007;47(5):697–704.

22. Simino BP, Feldman PH. ReACH National Demonstration Collaborative: early results of implementation. Home Health Care Serv Q 2007;26(4):105–20.

23. Rich MW, Beckham V, Wittenberg C, et al. A multidisciplinary intervention to prevent the readmission of elderly patients with congestive heart failure. N Engl J Med 1995;333:1190–5.

24. Naylor MD, Brooten D, Campbell R, et al. Comprehensive discharge planning and home care follow-up of hospitalized elders. JAMA 1999;281(7): 613–20.

25. Naylor MD, Brooten DA, Campbell RL, et al. Transitional care of older adults hospitalized with heart failure: a randomized, controlled trial. J Am Geriatr Soc 2004; 52(5):675–84.

26. Smigelski C, Hungate B, Holdren J, et al. Transitional model of care at VCU Medical Center – 6 years' experience. J Am Geriatr Soc 2008;65(4 Suppl):S197.

27. Phillips SL, Phillips JV, Branaman-Phillips J, et al. Geriatric versus non-geriatric approach of care to moderate Pra risk senior population. J Am Med Dir Assoc 2005;6(6):396–9.

28. Wennberg JE, Fisher ES, Goodman DC, et al. Tracking the care of patients with severe chronic illness. The Dartmouth Institute for Health Policy and Clinical Practice, Dartmouth College, ISBN 978-0-9815862-0-5; 2008. Available at: http://www. dartmouthatlas.org. Accessed December 18, 2008.

29. Newcomer R, Harrington C, Kane R. Implementing the second generation social health maintenance organization. J Am Geriatr Soc 2000;48(7):829–34.

30. Martin DC, Berger ML, Anstatt DT, et al. A randomized controlled open trial of population-based disease and case management in a Medicare Plus Choice health maintenance organization. Prev Chronic Dis 2004;1(4):1–11.

31. Hebert PL, Sisk JE, Wang JJ, et al. Cost-effectiveness of nurse-led disease management for heart failure in an ethnically diverse urban community. Ann Intern Med 2008;149(8):540–8.

32. Quinn JL, Prybylo M, Pannone P. Community care management across the continuum. Study results from a Medicare health maintenance plan. Care Manag J 1999;1(4):223–31.

33. Hughes SL, Weaver FM, Giobbie-Hurder A, et al. Department of Veterans Affairs Cooperative Study Group on Home-Based Primary Care. Effectiveness of team-managed home-based primary care: a randomized multicenter trial. JAMA 2000; 284(22):2877–85.

34. Kripalani S, Jackson AT, Schnipper JL, et al. Promoting effective transitions of care at hospital discharge: a review of key issues for hospitalists. J Hosp Med 2007;2:314–23.
35. Delate T, Chester EA, Stubbings TW, et al. Clinical outcomes of a home-based medication reconciliation program after discharge from a skilled nursing facility. Pharmacotherapy 2008;28(4):444–52.
36. Parry C, Mahoney E, Chalmers SA, et al. Assessing the quality of transitional care: further applications of the care transitions measure. Med Care 2008; 46(3):317–22.
37. Coleman EA, Parry C, Chalmers SA, et al. The central role of performance improvement in improving the quality of transitional care. Home Health Care Serv Q 2007;26(4):93–104.
38. Cigolle CT, Langa KM, Kabeto MU, et al. Setting eligibility criteria for a care-co-ordination benefit. J Am Geriatr Soc 2005;53(12):2051–9.

Veteran's Affairs Home Based Primary Care

Julie Leftwich Beales, MD, PhD, MSHA[a],*, Thomas Edes, MD, MS[b]

KEYWORDS

- Home care • Chronic disease
- Non-institutional long-term care • Interdisciplinary team
- Home based primary care

The changing demographics of the American population are a source of concern for health care economists and policymakers. The population of Americans older than 85 years is projected to increase 44% between the years 2000 and 2010. During these same 10 years, the number of veterans older than 85 years actually doubled in the first 5 years and is projected to nearly triple, increasing 190% by 2010.[1]

This means that the VA has been facing the challenges of a burgeoning older population a decade earlier and with a sharper increase than the rest of the nation. Fortunately, many bright and dedicated individuals within the VA anticipated this challenge and have been preparing the VA for the care of this elderly population for decades.

With the increase in aging population comes not only an increase in the numbers but also an increase in prevalence of associated disease and disability. Nearly half of all Americans older than 85 years are dependent in at least one activity of daily living. This includes bathing, dressing, toileting, transferring, and feeding. In addition, nearly half of Americans older than 85 years have dementia, greatly increasing the need for daily assistance. In response to these demographic changes, the VA created a spectrum of programs to provide services to this unique population. These programs are designed to meet the needs of individuals who are developing increasing complexity in their health care and impaired functional status. This article focuses on the VA's program called HBPC, a home care program that specifically targets individuals with complex chronic disabling disease, with the goal of maximizing the independence of the patient and reducing preventable emergency room visits and hospitalizations.

The costs of chronic disease are substantial, with two-thirds of Medicare dollars being spent on 10% of beneficiaries, most of whom have five or more chronic conditions. The VA turns to those with special expertise in the care of complex chronic disease, particularly individuals who have training and expertise in geriatrics. HBPC

[a] VAMC, 1201 Broad Rock Blvd, Richmond, VA 23249, USA
[b] Home and Community-Based Care, U.S. Department of Veterans Affairs, Washington, DC 20420, USA
* Corresponding author.
E-mail address: julie.beales@va.gov (J.L. Beales).

Clin Geriatr Med 25 (2009) 149–154
doi:10.1016/j.cger.2008.11.002
0749-0690/08/$ – see front matter. Published by Elsevier Inc.

geriatric.theclinics.com

targets patients with complex chronic disabling disease and uses an interdisciplinary team of these geriatric-skilled practitioners to provide comprehensive longitudinal primary care in the homes of veterans for whom routine clinic-based care is not effective. HBPC provides cost-effective primary care in the home, which may include palliative care, rehabilitation, disease management, and coordination of care.

The VA established the Hospital Based Home Care (HBHC) program with six sites in 1972. The program continued to add sites, but practice variations developed, including the degree of physician involvement in interventions and plan of care. In 1995, the VA changed the name of the program from Hospital Based Home Care (HBHC) to Home Based Primary Care (HBPC) and clarified the intent to deliver comprehensive primary care in the home. The new program standards delineate the responsibility for primary care, team composition and the roles of the interdisciplinary team's members, the selection criteria for the target population with advanced chronic diseases and disabilities, and the type and number of staff appropriate for the care of a specific number of patients. In the new HBPC model, HBPC becomes the primary care provider. This role is fulfilled by the HBPC medical director alone or in collaboration with a midlevel nurse practitioner or physician assistant. The frequency of physician home visits depends on the composition and structure of the team.[2]

It is important to understand the differences between HBPC and other home care systems. Notably, HBPC is different from and complementary to Medicare home health agency care. The differences are in the target population, in the processes of care, and in the outcomes (**Table 1**).

HBPC selectively targets individuals with complex chronic disease, whereas Medicare home care often serves persons with remediable and short-term conditions. HBPC provides comprehensive primary care, whereas Medicare home care is designed to provide problem-focused skilled care. HBPC is routinely provided through an interdisciplinary team; Medicare home care is generally provided by one provider or a series of individuals with relatively little team integration. HBPC often provides longitudinal care for months or years; Medicare home care is increasingly focused on episodic postacute care. HBPC is strongly associated with a reduction in inpatient days and total cost of care, whereas an extensive analysis of Medicare home care identified no significant impact on hospital days or total cost of care.[3-5]

HBPC provides longitudinal comprehensive interdisciplinary care to veterans with complex chronic disease. The HBPC population has a mean age of 76.5 years.

Table 1
Differences between VA HBPC and Medicare skilled home care

VA HBPC	Medicare Skilled Home Care
Targets chronic disease	Targets remediable conditions
Comprehensive primary care	Problem-focused care
Interdisciplinary team every time	One or multiple disciplines
Homebound not strictly required	Must be homebound
Skilled care not required	Requires skilled care need
Longitudinal care	Episodic, postacute care
Accepts declining status	Emphasizes improvement
Reduces hospital days	No definitive impact
Limited geography and intensity	Anywhere and anytime

Abbreviations: HBPC, Home Based Primary Care; VA, Department of Veterans Affairs.

Because this is an older veteran population they are 96% men; this predominance of men is shifting somewhat as there are more women in the newer generations of veterans. Of the patients enrolled in HBPC, 47% are dependent in two or more activities of daily living. Nearly half of the veterans in HBPC are married, and of those, one-third of the spousal caregivers have limitations in their activities of daily living. Therefore, the care of these veterans and maintaining them in their homes become progressively greater challenges. The HBPC veterans have a high prevalence of chronic disease, each having on average more than eight hierarchical chronic conditions. In 2007, 72% of the veterans had heart disease, 48% had diabetes, 35% had heart failure, and at least one-third had dementia. Another 29% had cancer, and nearly one in five had chronic lung disease. The HBPC population also has a high prevalence of stroke, with residual deficits, Parkinson's disease, and other neurologic conditions. HBPC is not restricted by age, and a substantial proportion of veterans have underlying neurologic disease, such as multiple sclerosis, that may make them appropriate candidates for HBPC at a relatively early age.[6,7]

Because of the population targeted and enrolled in HBPC, the goals are very different from those of skilled care in the home. Goals of care for HBPC patients as outlined in the 2007 Veterans Health Administration (VHA) HBPC Handbook are enumerated in the following list.

GOALS OF HBPC

1. Promoting the veteran's maximum level of health and independence by providing comprehensive care and optimizing physical, cognitive, and psychosocial functions.
2. Reducing the need for, and providing an acceptable alternative to, hospitalization, nursing home care, and emergency department and outpatient clinic visits, through longitudinal care that provides close monitoring, early intervention, and a therapeutic safe home environment.
3. Assisting in the transition from a health care facility to the home by providing patient and caregiver education, guiding rehabilitation and use of adaptive equipment in the home, adapting the home as needed for a safe and therapeutic environment, and arranging and coordinating supportive services, including home telehealth, as appropriate.
4. Supporting the caregiver in the care of the veteran.
5. Meeting the changing needs and preferences of the veteran and family throughout the course of chronic disease, often through the end of life.
6. Enhancing the veteran's quality of life through symptom management and other comfort measures.
7. Allowing the veteran the option of dying at home rather than in an institution.
8. Helping the veteran and family cope with all elements of chronic disease.
9. Promoting an enduring network of skilled home health care professionals by providing an academic and clinical setting for health care trainees to experience interdisciplinary delivery of primary care in the home.

As can be seen, these HBPC goals are all inclusive of care of the patient in the home to include close monitoring possibly using telehealth, a therapeutic safe home environment, support of the caregiver, palliative care, and the option of death at home. HBPC personnel are able to provide primary care, chronic disease management, physical therapy, social work intervention, nutrition management, home safety evaluation, ongoing case management, and, more recently, mental health services. Via collaboration with other VA programs, such as contracted skilled care, adult day health care programs, homemaker, home health aide, and home hospice, HBPC is able to help provide the patient and family with much needed services, which often make a difference in the patient being able to remain in the home. Briefly stated, HBPC meets the changing needs and preferences of the veteran and family throughout the course of chronic disease, often through the end of life.

Additional operational details distinguish HBPC from other models of home care. Veterans are enrolled in HBPC longitudinally, on average for more than 315 days, in contrast to Medicare home care, in which episodes of care average 65 days. HBPC patients average slightly more than three visits per month from the combination of all interdisciplinary team members. HBPC enrollment does not require a skilled care need, does not require strict homebound status, and can continue providing comprehensive home care despite declining status. Medicare home care requires a skilled care need, it serves only homebound persons, and, for continued rehabilitative therapy, there must be demonstration of progress toward a defined goal. Since HBPC targets individuals with complex chronic and progressively debilitating disease, many patients are not expected to improve, and they have continuous care needs often until the end of life. VA HBPC teams are successful if they slow the decline of these patients with advanced chronic diseases and allow them to remain in their homes as long as possible. HBPC is interdisciplinary, requires that teams meet regularly, and develops a single unified care plan for the team.

Because of the design of its services, HBPC is limited in geography and service intensity. HBPC programs have geographic restrictions because the team is based at a facility—generally a VA hospital. For that reason, the area of coverage tends to range 30 to 70 miles from the facility. Therefore, many areas in the country do not have coverage by HBPC. Additionally, if an individual needs home visits more than once a day or even multiple times a week for a prolonged period, the HBPC program cannot meet that intensity of service. Medicare home care can reach patients nearly anywhere and provide services at any time. Through the complementary nature of these programs, if a veteran needs services that are beyond the scope of the HBPC team, VA uses skilled services either through Medicare or through VA contract payment in a concurrent fashion with HBPC, being careful to avoid duplication of services.

HBPC uses a highly interdisciplinary approach involving a diverse array of professionals who are required to effectively manage the complex health problems of chronically or terminally ill patients. The core team is composed of a physician, nurses, social worker, rehabilitation therapist, pharmacist, dietitian, and recently a psychologist. The registered nurse functions as a case manager who continually assesses the patient's needs and delivers home nursing care. The midlevel provider has primary medical management responsibility in conjunction with the supervising physician. The social worker assesses interpersonal resources and relationships of the veteran, family, other caregivers, and their support systems and helps maximize available VA and non-VA resources. The dietitian performs ongoing assessment of nutritional status, recognizing the important role of nutrition in the management of chronic conditions, and provides individualized guidance to improve the patient's condition or prevent exacerbations. The rehabilitation therapist assesses functional status, evaluates the home for structural modifications needed to make the home safe and accessible, determines need for home medical equipment, and establishes a therapeutic program to maximize functional independence. The pharmacist assesses medication therapy; identifies adverse events, risks, discrepancies, noncompliance, and duplications; educates the veteran and caregiver regarding proper use of medications;

participates in team meetings; educates staff on medication interactions and uses; and recommends regimen changes.[3]

In 2002, the VA conducted a national analysis of the use of HBPC and cost for the veterans who received care in HBPC. This analysis compared the 6 months before enrollment in HBPC with the next 6 months during HBPC. The results from 11,334 veterans in HBPC included reduction in hospital bed days of care by 62%, reduction in nursing home bed days of care by 88%, and an increase in all home care visits by 264%. The mean total VA cost of care dropped 24%, from $38,000 to $29,000 per patient per year. Building on this study, in 2006 the VA implemented a quality measure for HBPC that continually assesses the impact of HBPC on reducing inpatient use, comparing VA hospital and nursing home use during HBPC to the 6 months before enrollment in HBPC.

Enrollment in HBPC for fiscal year 2007, was associated with a 59% reduction in hospital bed days of care, an 89% reduction in nursing home bed days of care, and a combined reduction of 78% in total inpatient days of care. Enrollment in HBPC was also associated with a 21% reduction in 30-day hospital readmission rates. Notably, the 79% reduction in total inpatient days is greater than the 29% reduction in inpatient admissions. This difference implies that HBPC is effective not only at reducing the frequency of hospitalizations but also at shortening the length of hospital stays. The VA is in the process of determining which factors have the strongest association with reduction in inpatient days. While further analysis continues, the initial findings indicate that the specific program characteristics that are linked with the greatest reduction in inpatient days include targeting individuals with multiple comorbidities and multiple prior hospitalizations, home visits by the HBPC team physician, nurse practitioner, or physician assistant, interdisciplinary team experience, and smaller caseloads.[8,9]

The VA recognizes that there is a high prevalence of mental illness and behavioral conditions among the veteran population in HBPC. Of HBPC patients, 44% have depression, 29% have substance abuse, 24% have anxiety or personality disorder, 21% have posttraumatic stress disorder, and 20% have schizophrenia.[2] Each of these conditions greatly adds complexity to the effective management of individuals with chronic disease. It is critically important that mental health is addressed in the overall management of individuals with chronic disease. As a result of this recognition VA established mental health positions in HBPC and now has a mental health provider, generally a psychologist, in every HBPC program in the country. Many programs are adding more mental health staff because of the prevalence of mental disease and the great demand for their services. These mental health providers routinely make home visits and are an integral part of the interdisciplinary team. It is believed that this is an important aspect of home care for persons with complex chronic disabling disease, and it is sought to establish this as a standard of practice in home care for all health care systems.

The Congressional Budget Office (CBO) published a report in December 2007 on the costs of health care from 1998 through 2005, comparing costs within VA to costs under Medicare.[8] In these 7 years, the annual cost of health care per patient within the VA rose 1.7% or 0.3% per year, whereas the cost within Medicare rose 29% or 4.4% per year. The CBO identified the highest cost sectors to be those with patients who had advanced chronic disease and were homebound. They suggested that the three factors most likely to contribute to VA's success in controlling health care costs were (1) the electronic medical record; (2) the system being driven strongly by quality and performance measures; and (3) programs that are specifically designed for the management of chronic disabling disease. VA HBPC is one of these programs.

Home care for chronic disease is not effective as an episodic inoculation. Effective home care for persons with complex chronic disease must be comprehensive, not problem-focused. It must be longitudinal, not episodic. It must be interdisciplinary, not delivered by one or two providers. Moreover, it must integrate primary care. If complex chronic disabling disease is the question, home care is the answer, and the VA HBPC experience now provides the United States with substantial evidence to support this view.

REFERENCES

1. VetPop2004. Available at: http://www1.va.gov/vetdata/docs/VP2004B.htm. Accessed August 16, 2008.
2. VHA Handbook 1141.01. Home-based primary care program. Available at: http://vaww1.va.gov/vhapublications. Accessed January 31, 2007.
3. Welch HG, Wennberg DE, Welch WP. The use of medicare home health care services. N Engl J Med 1996;335:324–9.
4. Dartmouth Atlas. Tracking the care of patients with severe chronic illness. Available at: http://www.dartmouthatlas.org/atlases/2008_Chronic_Care_Atlas.pdf. 2008. Accessed October 27, 2008.
5. Edes T, Tompkins H. Quality measure of reduction of inpatient days during Home Based Primary Care (HBPC). J Am Geriatr Soc 2007;55(4, Suppl):S7.
6. US Department of Veterans Affairs. Veterans Health Administration VISN Support Service Center (VSSC). Veterans Affairs; 2008.
7. Austin VA. HBPC Database—an internal VA database.
8. Percy A, Gilmore JM, Goldberg MS. The health care system for veterans: an interim report. Congressional Budget Office. Available at: http://www.cbo.gov/ftpdocs/88xx/doc8892/12-21-VA_Healthcare.pdf. December, 2007. Accessed October 27, 2008.
9. Kinosian B, Tompkins H, Edes T. Factors associated with reduction in inpatient days by Home Based Primary Care (HBPC). J Am Geriatr Soc 2008;65(Suppl 4): S197–8.

Independence at Home: Community-Based Care for Older Adults with Severe Chronic Illness

K. Eric DeJonge, MD[a],*, George Taler, MD[a], Peter A. Boling, MD[b]

KEYWORDS

- Home care • Home health care • House calls
- Health care financing • Health policy
- Cost effectiveness • Health care reform

The well-being of the US health care system depends on how well we manage a growing and costly population of older patients with severe chronic illness and disability. Medicare was designed in 1965 to prevent financial ruin when elders needed basic hospital care. This occurred before the emergence of many costly procedures and drugs that now sustain older persons through years of advanced chronic illness.

Until recently, health care has relied heavily on an acute care paradigm designed to handle brief episodes of illness. However, the growing number of elders with advanced chronic illness has become a major driver of morbidity and Medicare costs.[1,2] In this article, we review prior efforts to improve care for elders with severe chronic illness, assess why these efforts have often failed to improve outcomes or save money, and propose an alternative model, called independence at home (IAH). IAH addresses Medicare's root problems: poorly coordinated care and incentives to perform large volumes of procedural care regardless of clinical or economic outcome.

Who are the highest-cost Medicare beneficiaries? We know that 5% of the Medicare population (approximately 2 million people) consume nearly half of the Medicare budget (**Fig. 1**).[2] We also know that functional disability predicts higher medical costs.[3] Finally, although some patients develop a single catastrophic illness from which they recover fully or die, most patients with multiple chronic illnesses have a high likelihood of being persistent high-cost users over a period of several years.[2] This combination of facts paints a picture: a small subgroup of Medicare beneficiaries

[a] Section of Geriatrics and Long-Term Care, Washington Hospital Center, 110 Irving Street NW, Washington, DC 20010, USA
[b] Department of Internal Medicine, Virginia Commonwealth University, PO Box 980102, Richmond, VA 23298, USA
* Corresponding author.
E-mail address: karl.e.dejonge@medstar.net (K.E. DeJonge).

Clin Geriatr Med 25 (2009) 155–169
doi:10.1016/j.cger.2008.11.004
0749-0690/08/$ – see front matter © 2009 Elsevier Inc. All rights reserved.

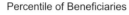

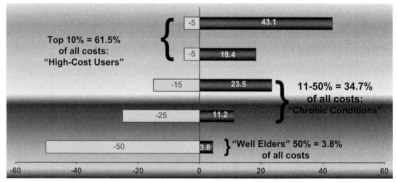

Fig. 1. Annual Medicare expenditures among beneficiaries, 2001. (*Data from* United States Congressional Budget Office. High-cost Medicare beneficiaries. Washington DC, 2005.)

with multiple chronic illnesses, functional disability, and history of high prior use drive about half of the Medicare budget.

It is vital to distinguish this subgroup of very ill individuals from the much larger population of functional elders with one or two chronic diseases such as asthma, diabetes, arthritis, or hypertension. This latter group has been estimated to include up to 20 million Medicare beneficiaries and is the focus of disease management (DM) programs.[4] The very high-cost beneficiaries, those with multiple severe illnesses and dependence on others for care, are a very different population.

These very high-cost elders usually have several chronic illnesses, such as heart failure, vascular disease, stroke, diabetes, hypertension, chronic obstructive pulmonary disease, renal disease, and dementia, which are confounded by psychological stress, financial hardship, social upheaval, and legal problems. These factors greatly increase the complexity of their care. These persons often live for years while disabled and in poor health. Their illnesses put them at high risk for hospitalization. Their frequent use of hospitals, nursing homes, and home health care place them into the highest-cost group. In a study of high-cost users in 2001 who lived for 5 years, the median survivor was in a high-cost category during 22 out of 60 months.[2] Approximately 2 million persons (5% of Medicare beneficiaries) have multiple chronic illnesses and disability and would likely benefit from coordination of medical, social, and housing services.[5]

While primary medical and social services, when well-coordinated, often have a favorable impact on health for at-risk elders, they are not rewarded by the present reimbursement system. Instead, Medicare payments encourage providers to maximize the volume of specialty procedures and acute care, which increases care fragmentation, risks of complications, and overall costs.

Recent evidence shows that the use of subspecialty and acute care services are "supply-sensitive." This means that consumption is influenced by the number of specialty physicians, high-tech devices, or hospital beds per capita in a region, rather than by patients' needs. This leads to a marked regional variation in Medicare spending, with no discernible difference in health outcomes and suggests that much Medicare spending fails to benefit patients.[6] The Dartmouth Atlas project and Congressional Budget Office (CBO) have estimated that a 30% cost reduction is feasible for Medicare without compromising health outcomes.[2,6] It is worth noting that services such as reperfusion for acute heart attacks, joint replacement surgery, and mammograms are evenly distributed by region. Medical provider visits, diagnostic tests, and inpatient hospital days show the most regional variation.[1]

Since many high-cost patients are immobile and best served at home, we will concentrate on models of care for these chronically ill patients. The main approaches to their care as described by Murkofsky, Leff, Newcomer and others elsewhere in this issue are split into two conceptual frames: (1) post-acute care funded by Medicare and private payers and (2) chronic supportive care funded by Medicaid and out-of-pocket expenses. Although the patient's home was not envisioned as a primary locus of care when Medicare was enacted, the home is often the preferred setting for care of ill elders, and in many cases, it is the least expensive and safest.[7] We argue that reform of health care delivery for high-cost elders should include incentives to offer comprehensive care in the community, both for the welfare of vulnerable patients and for the societal pocketbook.

EVOLUTION OF CHRONIC CARE MODELS

The US population's aging demography, modern medicine's success in preventing death from acute illness, the growing prevalence of severe chronic illness, and a desire to lessen institutional care have motivated attempts to redesign health care for high-risk elders. In the past 20 years, the United States has explored several alternative models of care and financing. These include the social health maintenance organization (S/HMO), PACE, Medicare Care Coordination (MCC) demo, Special Needs Program (SNP), Chronic Care Model (CCM), Medicare Health Support (MHS), Disease Management (DM) and, most recently, the Advanced Medical Home (AMH).

These models have revised certain aspects of elder care and have had limited success, but none has created a community-based, mobile system of care that rewards better clinical and economic outcomes for the most high-cost Medicare patients. Unfortunately, these efforts have failed to stem a sharp decline in the supply of primary care physicians for elders and have not fostered the development of more geriatricians.

Social Health Maintenance Organizations

The S/HMO model was introduced in 1985. This was a Medicare managed care product that combined risk-based financing under capitation with additional chronic care services, such as care coordination, short-term respite care, drug coverage, homemaker services, and adult day care. These extras were covered by an augmented Medicare payment, based on a rate adjusted for patient severity and complexity.

In the "S/HMO I" era (1985–1996), four demonstration sites originated in facility-based organizations. S/HMOs did not engage physicians in the care plan and did not have the intended effects on resource use.[8] The S/HMO program evaluation noted lower patient satisfaction than that in fee-for-service beneficiaries and similar satisfaction compared with that in other Medicare managed care plans. There was no decrease in overall costs and no notable improvement in patients' health or function. The S/HMO II era (1996–1999) used a revised approach that incorporated primary care physicians and geriatric care concepts, but only one of the original four S/HMOs continued as an S/HMO II organization, and no other companies chose to replicate the model.

The final verdict was that S/HMOs "have not proven they are worth the substantial additional cost to Medicare."[8] In 2001, the government phased the S/HMO program into the Medicare-Plus-Choice managed care program and reduced their payments. These managed care plans have selectively recruited healthier elders and focused management strategies for patients with chronic illnesses on moving patients aggressively from hospitals to post-acute care settings. Ambulatory patients with more complex care needs were marginalized and tended to drop out. The S/HMOs ultimately closed, because the beneficiaries they were designed to attract and their chronic care costs made the organizations noncompetitive.

Program for All-Inclusive Care of the Elderly

Another model of care for frail elders is PACE. PACE was pioneered in San Francisco in the early 1970s, when a Chinatown-North Beach community identified the long-term care needs of immigrant ethnic Chinese. The community leaders formed a nonprofit corporation, On Lok Senior Health Services, to create a community-based system of elder care.[9]

The core principle of PACE is that seniors with chronic care needs are best served in the community. PACE financing is risk-based using capitation; PACE programs receive combined funds from Medicare and Medicaid plus some Housing and Urban Development dollars. PACE serves individuals who are 55 years or older, are eligible for Medicare and Medicaid, and are certified as nursing home eligible but able to live in the community. PACE sites provide a continuum of services to elders with chronic care needs (**Table 1**).[9]

The PACE hub is an adult day center where enrollees socialize and receive medical and social services. PACE funding is determined by average Medicare and Medicaid regional expenses for a given group, defined by sex, 5-year age bracket, and a diagnosis-based cost profile. PACE participants are a low-income group (Medicaid-eligible) and must be eligible for nursing home care, but only 7% of participants actually live in a nursing home, suggesting that this model does keep frail elders in the community.

PACE was made a permanent federal health benefit in 1997. By 2007, there were 42 PACE sites in 22 states, with most sites having 100–200 participants, and 15,000 individuals enrolled nationwide overall.[9] To date, PACE programs have provided high-quality services, demonstrated improved function in some sites, kept most enrollees

Table 1
PACE core services[9]
Primary medical care by PACE physician and/or nurse practitioner
Adult day care at the PACE center
Medical specialty care
Hospital and nursing home care
Home health and personal care
Physical, occupational, and recreational therapies
Nursing care
Social work services
Nutritional counseling
Prescription drug coverage
Respite services

out of nursing homes, and have been generally fiscally healthy. Reasons for slow adoption of the PACE model include strict clinical and income entry criteria and reluctance of health systems to invest several million dollars of capital to establish the adult day care center and escrow funds needed for the financial risk model.[10]

Notably, PACE sites with higher hospitalization rates have reported worse risk-adjusted functional outcomes, suggesting that it may be safer for such patients to stay out of the hospital.[11] Other PACE evaluations found that a few sites have enrolled populations with higher functional status and lower disease burden, and there is variation in the service models between the sites.[12,13] In the final analysis, although PACE is an excellent care model, PACE has served a small number of frail elders and has not demonstrated overall cost savings for Medicare and Medicaid.[14]

Chronic Care Model

Another approach is the chronic care model (CCM), developed by Wagner and colleagues in the mid-1990s in collaboration with the Robert Wood Johnson Foundation (RWJF).[15–17] CCM originated with a finding that when caring for patients with chronic illness, clinicians often do not follow evidence-based guidelines or provide care coordination, and patients are not trained to manage their own illness. The CCM defines elements needed to improve chronic care at the community, organization, practice, and patient level. This involves self-management, delivery system redesign, and clinical information systems. The core idea is to promote evidence-based change in office-based care.[18]

In 2003, the CCM was updated to focus on patient safety, cultural competency, care coordination, and case management. Some view CCM as a primary care model and not a DM approach, but the setting remains the physician office, and the emphasis is on management of specific diseases, such as asthma or diabetes, rather than disabled patients with multiple chronic illnesses.[19] An RWJF report on the CCM Web site notes challenges with changing the behaviors of office-based physicians and health organizations and that execution of CCM principles requires a substantial increase in provider time and expense.[20]

Some data suggest that CCM care can save $500 to $1,000/y on the care of a person with diabetes.[21] However, we found no evidence that CCM reduces costs of care for elders with multiple chronic illnesses and functional disability. The CCM model is an effort to standardize office-based ambulatory care but applies less well to the highest-cost individuals who generate most of the annual growth in costs.[22] Furthermore, the CCM approach is office-based, which applies less well to very ill and disabled elders.

Special Needs Plans

In 2003, Medicare created the SNPs within Medicare Advantage. An SNP identifies beneficiaries in certain subsets of the population with anticipated high costs, including: (1) institutionalized persons; (2) Medicare and Medicaid dually eligible persons in the community; and (3) beneficiaries with severe or disabling chronic conditions. SNPs enroll Medicare patients of all ages, not just 65 years and older, and provide extra services to improve quality of care. Monthly payments are per capita, based on Medicare payments for the region, and managed by Medicare Advantage plans, which take risk for all Medicare-covered expenses.

It is too early to assess the full impact of SNPs, but in early 2008, initial data did not show the clinical or economic benefits envisioned and raised uncertainty about whether SNPs would continue. A possible weakness of SNPs is the breadth of inclusion criteria, which means they may not always focus on high-cost beneficiaries with multiple chronic illnesses and disability. Several decades of health service research show that targeting the highest-risk and highest-cost subgroups is the key to saving money.[23]

Another potential problem is that some SNPs operate within HMO (Health Management Organization) reimbursement and care delivery systems, which can be less attractive to patients and providers. In addition, fees and subsidies paid to Medicare Advantage plans and SNPs were lessened in 2008, which may lessen the viability of this business model.

Medicare Health Support

In 2003, Medicare created the Voluntary Chronic Care Improvement (VCCI) pilot program, since renamed medicare health support (MHS). This program assigned 20,000 elders with one or more chronic illnesses to large organizations, most of which were disease management (DM) organizations, and held them responsible for clinical and economic outcomes.[24] Most MHS organizations did not provide in-person medical care and focused on phone-based DM.

Care Level Management (CLM), perhaps the most promising of the MHS organizations, made routine and urgent house calls as its signature service, but CLM existed in parallel with patients' office-based medical providers. In the CLM demonstration, providers were assigned thousands of patients, most already under the care of other physicians, and attempted to recruit them into the CLM comanagement program. This contrasts with the preferred approach of growing a primary care service from a community base and responding directly to the needs of patients and families. This design made success unlikely, and the Secretary of HHS (Health and Human Services) terminated MHS in July 2008 due to lack of cost savings.[25]

Disease Management

In the past 15 years, there has been a proliferation of disease-specific clinical approaches to chronic diseases, under the rubric of "DM." The basic DM principle is conceptually sound: in an environment where compliance with care guidelines is inconsistent, applying evidence-based care to patients with chronic disease may improve outcomes. Yet, despite the billions of dollars invested to date, there is a remarkable paucity of evidence that DM has either saved money or improved outcomes, as noted in a 2002 report to Congress by the CBO.[26] More recently, Center for Medicare and Medicaid (CMS) analysts commented that DM was not a success for Medicare, mainly on the basis of the MHS demonstration described above, and that other approaches to chronic illness care should be sought.[27,28] This conclusion is not surprising. Improved outcomes from DM, which are best-used in a moderate risk population, if they occur at all, take years to materialize. The highest-cost care is driven by patients with multiple, severe chronic illnesses and disability, not by ambulatory elders with 1 or 2 chronic diseases.

Advanced Medical Home

Most recently, the advanced medical home (AMH) has been promoted by many major physician organizations and on Capitol Hill. The AMH idea is that any patient with a chronic illness should have a "medical home," meaning an enhanced physician's office.[29] In many respects, the AMH model follows CCM principles and designs, but it has the benefit of a monthly per-beneficiary reimbursement for eligible patients, to offset additional costs to the practice and to enhance the provider's income.

The AMH aims to encourage patient-centered, physician-guided, and efficient care. A primary physician helps patients navigate the health care system with plans customized to the patients' needs. Most patients use a primary care AMH physician, but a specialist's office may serve as an AMH for patients with certain dominant conditions (eg, severe asthma, severe diabetes, complicated cardiovascular disease, rheumatologic disorders, or malignancies). To qualify as a Tier two AMH and an even higher level of reimbursement, a physician practice must offer 19 specific services, including care coordination, DM, and electronic health records (EHR).[30]

Unfortunately, the AMH suffers from nonspecific patient entry criteria, which means that up to 86% of Medicare beneficiaries would be eligible based on having 1 or more of 283 eligible diagnoses. In addition, the AMH does not hold providers accountable for clinical outcomes or overall savings. Although the AMH model rewards qualified physician practices with an extra monthly payment, it excludes from the payment model other health providers who care for ill elders (eg, hospitals, nursing homes, and home care agencies).

In summary, the AMH does not focus on the most ill patients, does not change the primary setting of care for high-cost and disabled elders from physician office to the home, and does not require overall cost savings. The care of disabled elders in the AMH model would rely heavily on interventions by home health nurses and telemedicine rather than by direct medical staff. A focus on care of persons with severe chronic illness is expected to occur in later stages of AMH development, but it would involve a small fraction of the patients in a typical medical practice. From the outset, the AMH model requires substantial investment in new office infrastructure, which will be available to more mobile and lower-cost elders. This raises questions about the ability of the AMH model to save money on the highest-cost elders. The results from the AMH demonstration project are due in 2013.[30]

THE CLINICAL CHALLENGE

A major health care challenge is the leading edge of the baby boom: the first of these people turn 65 in 2011. By 2020, the number of elders in the United States will increase from 36 to 50 million.[31] The fastest growing group, however, are those aged 85 years and older, who will nearly double in number from four million to more than seven million by 2020. These old-old persons have the greatest burden of severe chronic illness, functional disability, and fragile social support systems. Technical advances in medical care have transformed the final chapters of their lives from acute illness and rapid death to recurrent exacerbations of chronic illness and a slow death, after years of increasing frailty. We have not yet adapted our health care systems to their needs.

For these ill and frail elders, we assert that most primary care should occur in the home, with coordinated efforts to address social issues, functional disability, and intensive medical management.[32] The care should focus on improving symptoms and comfort and less on acute care, technical services, and a quixotic quest for disease "cures." The familiar surrounding of home with family and friends is often a safer, less expensive, and a preferred setting for care. Very ill elders cannot get to the office in a timely way when they are sick and, once there, a typical office lacks the social, nursing, and supportive services that such patients need. Additionally, transitions in and out of institutional care settings are fraught with peril as discussed by Boling elsewhere in this issue.

A successful model of care for very ill elders must address more than medical care of selected diseases. To provide the holistic care, we must change the delivery system from a doctor-centered office setting to a mobile approach centered in the elder's home. The PACE model does this to some degree, but the entry criteria, financing (Medicaid eligibility), and organizational structure requirements are too restrictive to scale up for a larger Medicare population. Hospice is also an excellent service model but addresses care only in the final months of life. The human and societal costs of severe chronic illness predate this terminal phase of illness by several years, and hospice care is too expensive to sustain for such an extended period in most cases.

In sum, many of the CCMs reviewed thus far do not get at the root of our broken health care delivery system. Although each has valuable attributes, most require the sick elder to come to the doctor, rather than organizing care where the frail elder lives and providing timely response when they get unsafe or sick.

THE THREATS

Respected authorities view rising combined costs of Medicare and Medicaid as the most serious federal budget concern.[33] The need to contain Medicare costs has led to a series of proposed provider fee cuts. Over a 10-year period, the 1997 Balanced Budget Act produced a planned reduction of $400 billion in provider payments. Medicare hospital spending growth saw a sustained plateau after implementing the diagnosis-related group payment in the 1980s, and home health care spending declined sharply following changes in payment in the late 1990s. Medicare payment pressures have caused hospitals to discharge patients aggressively to post-acute care settings with substandard continuity of care and pressured office providers to see more patients per hour. The arrival of the baby boom cohort is a concern, but the more serious problem is rising Medicare costs per capita, which far exceeds the annual rate of inflation.

Despite recent Medicare payment cuts, the Medicare budget continues its unabated growth: $454 billion in FY08 is slated to jump 10% to $499 billion in FY09. At this pace, one decade from now, in 2018, Medicare annual costs could reach $900 billion. With no corresponding additional revenues, experts anticipate dissolution of the Medicare Hospital Insurance Trust Fund before 2018.[34] At that point, Medicare Part A annual expenses of several hundred billion dollars would have to be covered by general tax revenues. The Government Accountability Office (GAO) views the Medicare cost projections as the single greatest threat to long-term stability of the federal budget.[34] Long-term spending for Medicare and Medicaid is a more serious fiscal challenge than Social Security, and, by 2050, it will have risen from 4% to 12% of the gross domestic product, while Social Security costs will increase from 4.3% to 6.1% of the GDP.[35] These inflation-adjusted numbers have the attention of all policy makers.

Serious consequences follow. The budgetary pressures from Medicare fee cuts threaten the integrity of the doctor–patient relationship by reducing the time per visit and jeopardizing patient safety during transitions between settings of care. Lower salaries, higher debt, and loss of professional satisfaction have a chilling effect on physicians entering primary care. Recent graduates specialize, focus on hospital medicine, seek concierge practice outside of Medicare, or leave clinical medicine altogether. Few pursue geriatric careers, and the number of geriatricians is declining as the population of elders is rising as discussed by Hiyashi and colleagues elsewhere in this issue.

The Association of American Medical Colleges (AAMC) has declared an overall physician workforce shortage and recommended a 30% increase in medical school enrollees by 2015.[36] However, other experts note that the workforce problem involves maldistribution by region and specialty rather than an overall shortage of physicians.[37] Ultimately, a lack of primary care physicians and geriatricians will mean that elders with multiple chronic illnesses will remain in the hands of committees of specialist physicians, none of whom is responsible for the whole patient. This leads to a spiral of cost increases, reflexive payment cuts, and a continued decline of primary care.

Unless we redesign health care delivery for high-cost Medicare patients, we face unpleasant alternatives. One is to shift Medicare beneficiaries into private sector insurance programs, using an undefined mechanism to deter cherry picking. However, private payers rely on contracts with the existing systems that provide fragmented care and have little expertise in the care of elders with advanced chronic illness. Creating many different models inside thousands of insurance organizations with high overhead and limited experience in chronic care will be inefficient and not produce care that patients need or want.

In the near term, we face reduced Medicare payments to providers, including a planned 21% professional fee cut in January 2010. History suggests that this cut is not politically feasible. In July 2008, following an acrimonious debate, Congressional supermajorities overrode President Bush's veto to avert a 10.6% physician fee cut. If professional fees are not cut, a second possibility is to reduce services, which is also politically untenable. A third option is a steep hike in premiums and taxes, which may be the most unlikely political choice of all. Given these hurdles, we need effective new clinical models that generate short and long-term savings.

To end this litany on a positive note, in the past decade, there is evidence from several sources to suggest that improved care and substantial reductions in costs are possible using comprehensive care in the patient's home, if efforts focus on the most ill individuals. The documented savings range from 30% to 50% of total costs, as described by Boling, Beales, and Kao elsewhere in this issue. These result from the combined clinical benefits of comprehensive geriatric assessment in the home as demonstrated by Counsell[38] and others plus the clinical ability to respond urgently in a mobile fashion to patients' and effectively to changing health conditions.

THE INDEPENDENCE AT HOME (IAH) MODEL

We propose a new model of care for seriously ill elders, based on hundreds of house call programs now operating in the United States. The central core is a mobile team of primary medical, nursing, and social work staff who deliver comprehensive primary care to the patient's home. It is a patient-centered approach called IAH. This model addresses the desire of most seniors to age in place by changing the primary setting of care from institutions and offices to the home. It redirects payment from providers who perform high volumes of expensive procedural services to teams that improve the overall care of a well-defined ill and disabled population and achieve cost savings.[39]

Mobile, interdisciplinary IAH teams would replace office-based providers for the small subgroup of ill elders who are poorly served in the office setting. The teams offer access to care for sick homebound patients who have little or inadequate ongoing primary medical care due to their immobility. Typical IAH teams deliver and coordinate services in the home and across settings, including hospitals and nursing homes, where care is delivered by the primary IAH staff team or by the facility-based groups that work closely with the IAH team. The mobile, primary care IAH team serves as the hub of a wheel of services, most of which are home-based. The IAH staff coordinate all "spokes" of care, including acute and specialty medical services, home nursing, rehabilitation, pharmacy, medical equipment, home health aides, and hospice care. This network of community providers comes from existing community resources and are recruited to support the IAH patients and team. The IAH team also arranges legal and financial services when the need arises.

Each IAH team has as its team leader a credentialed, experienced primary care medical provider (physician or nurse practitioner), social work staff, and office support staff to handle phone calls, paperwork, and communications. Among other duties, all staff must pay attention to geographic scheduling to minimize travel time and maximize efficiency. To facilitate timely and accurate diagnosis and treatment, IAH medical staff members use portable technology to perform tests and treatments for a variety of conditions. Capital investment in mobile technology is modest, and operational cost is low, compared with facility-based care.

Many types of organizations could sponsor IAH teams, including hospitals, group medical practices, home care agencies, long-term care systems, or managed care systems. The key is less the base of operations and more the proper personnel and care delivery model. In the rapidly evolving context of financing care of people with severe chronic illness, many different types of organizations may see strategic benefit in creating an IAH care team.

The IAH model addresses the primary reasons that prior CCMs have failed. First, the IAH model changes the main care setting from institutions to the home. This offers better clinical information to the provider and allows a care team to intervene in a timely manner at the home, and avert costly medical and social crises that an office-based physician hears about when the patient is in the emergency room (ER). The mobile team prevents avoidable ER visits and hospitalizations by bringing clinical expertise and mobile technology to the home when clinical instability is first developing and treats many of these problems in the home. Finally, a home-based primary care team builds trust with an elder and their family over time, to help navigate the difficult final years of life with appropriate use of acute and specialty care while forgoing ineffective and expensive services.

Elements for Success

To keep elders at home, a mobile IAH team must be interdisciplinary and take responsibility for coordinating care across settings and time, throughout the patient's life. This requires committed administrative and clinical leadership and a qualified clinical staff. The medical staff should be certified in geriatrics or have substantial home care experience. All team members must have the clinical competencies, communication skills, willingness, and personality styles needed to treat frail elders. The IAH team must provide 24/7 access to knowledgeable on-call medical staff, triage and dispatch capacity, and an EHR with remote access. Through prompt clinical intervention, in concert with a patient's preferences, ER visits and hospitalizations can often be avoided or at least more efficiently managed.

A mature IAH team uses a wireless and interoperable EHR with access for internal and external providers. The EHR includes an electronic quality audit system, clinical decision support, patient tracking, billing, and financial reporting features. As described by Bayne elsewhere in this issue, because current wireless EHR technology is limited by data transfer speeds and standards, a basic EHR can meet initial needs of an IAH team as long as it has functional remote access.

Challenges for the IAH Model

Building and sustaining IAH teams require skilled and dedicated staff. One must recruit and retain qualified physicians or nurse practitioners to lead the teams. They must be compassionate and motivated to care for ill elders who are complex and approaching life's end. Though there are now relatively few such providers in the field, with strong financial incentives this can change. There is no shortage of altruism and willingness to serve among those entering the medical field, and there are examples of rapid workforce development in new medical fields. Two examples are palliative care services, supported by hospitals and hospices, and the hospitalist movement. In the late 1990s, there were fewer than 1,000 identified hospitalists, and in 2006, there were 20,000.[40] By 2010, some experts estimate there will be as many as 30,000 hospitalists. Flexible schedules, higher salaries, and a supportive work environment are keys to such rapid workforce growth. This same approach can be used to create a mobile geriatrics primary care workforce.

Strong staff support is vital to mitigating strain on IAH clinicians. Patients and caregivers are often distraught as they cope with the effects of severe chronic illness. Much staff work, such as tedious phone calls and paperwork, goes into coordinating the array of services needed for home-based care. These include home health agencies, Medicare Part D drug plan issues, social services, medical equipment, subspecialty care, information retrieval when patients are hospitalized, and arranging inpatient care or unavoidable changes in living situation.

IAH and other models of chronic care such as PACE depend on established services now present in most communities. As discussed by Murkofsky, Newcomer, and Brummel-Smith, elsewhere in this issue, the extensive architecture and workforce of nurses, therapists, pharmacists, social workers, aides, and medical device providers requires sustenance and integration. These organizations and their workforce are critical to the evolution of successful community-based care models.

Finally, there is a need to educate hospitals, physicians, community partners, and payers about the value of home-based medical care. The IAH model may be clinically effective, but it is unfamiliar to traditional health care providers.

Health Policy Change

Given the failure of some prior CCMs and the dire Medicare budget projections, there is a pressing need for successful models that achieve clinical and economic effectiveness. The Independence at Home (IAH) Act, introduced in the US Senate and House in September 2008 (H.R. 7114 and S. 3613) can accomplish these goals (Personal Communication. Pyles J. Powers, Pyles, Sutter, Verville, Inc. Independence at Home (IAH) Act (S. 3613, H.R. 7114). Beginning Medicare reform with the highest cost beneficiaries with the greatest need. Oct. 21, 2008.). The IAH Act provisions are as follows:

1. Mobile teams that provide coordinated home-based care to Medicare beneficiaries with multiple chronic illnesses, functional disability, and prior high health care costs.
2. IAH teams must show a minimum annual savings of 5% for Medicare, relative to predicted costs for the population served.
3. IAH providers to keep 80% of Medicare savings beyond the first 5% saved, to invest in information or mobile technology, staff development, and other clinical services that prevent high-cost events.
4. IAH providers are accountable for three minimum performance standards: patient and family satisfaction, good clinical outcomes, and the annual 5% savings.
5. IAH preserves all existing traditional Medicare coverage.
6. IAH preserves freedom of choice by making participation voluntary and allows elders to change IAH programs at any time.
7. IAH provides access to education and support for families and caregivers.

The IAH Act incorporates lessons learned from prior CCMs and from currently operating house call programs to improve care for ill elders. It promotes better care through a self-funded program and generates savings that can be used for other purposes by Congress. The IAH Act reforms the 1965 Medicare model to meet the clinical needs of frail elders now living in our communities.

Benefits of Funding Better Health Care Through Savings

The IAH program is based on a finding noted by the CBO that a small percentage reduction in the spending on the highest-cost beneficiaries could lead to large savings for the Medicare program. CBO noted that health care spending could be cut by up to 30% if the more conservative practice styles used in the lowest-spending one-fifth of the country were adopted.[2]

By using a shared savings payment rather than risk-based financing, IAH avoids the capitalization and strict enrollment criteria that slowed the growth of PACE. IAH organizations have the option of accepting no initial pay increase or taking a flat monthly fee for comprehensive geriatric assessments and coordination of the overall care plan. Any IAH organization that fails to achieve the 5% annual savings will keep all of their Medicare fee-for-service payments but must refund any monthly IAH payments received during the year, until all extra payments are returned or the 5% minimum savings is achieved, whichever comes first.

The IAH Act presents an opportunity to improve quality of care for our most ill elders. There is little risk to beneficiaries because they relinquish no benefits, can disenroll at any time, and can switch programs up to twice per year. There is limited risk to providers because only those who believe they can achieve savings will participate, and they are at risk only for the extra fees received during the year. Providers have strong incentives to select high-cost patients for IAH, who have more potential for cost savings, and to work hard at keeping them out of the hospital. There is minimal risk for Medicare, because IAH providers are accountable for a minimum 5% annual savings before any extra payments are made. Further, the government can terminate agreements of providers who do not meet the three core performance standards. This facilitates a comparative effectiveness process under which high-quality programs expand and poor-quality programs are eliminated.

The IAH model is achievable. It is built on demonstrated success of the nationwide Veterans' Affairs Home-Based Primary Care program, now with 130 sites and on hundreds of US house call programs that have been making home visits and saving Medicare dollars for years. Working with these experienced providers, and national organizations such as the American Academy of Home Care Physicians that have produced educational programs, books, ethics and clinical standards, and a forum for development, rapid growth is possible.

Importantly, the IAH Act will create incentives to expand the geriatrics workforce. Similar to the recent growth in the hospitalist workforce, based on the need for more efficient acute care, there is a need for more efficient elder care provided at home. This requires a new payment mechanism to draw physicians and other professionals into the field. With the revenues from shared savings, IAH providers can offer more generous salaries and lifestyle choices to geriatricians and other staff. IAH programs offer an enjoyable practice environment with portable technology and a capable interdisciplinary team. The opportunity to practice medicine well and to earn a competitive salary could help fill the sparsely populated ranks of primary care for elders in the community. Since the needs of the most complex older patients present the greatest economic and operational risk to office-based primary care, IAH should also help mainstream office-based care providers.

IAH teams will similarly draw more nurse practitioners, social workers, rehabilitation therapists, nurses, and home health aides into the field. The same rewards for excellent team-based care and better income will bring more professionals and paraprofessionals into elder care.

SUMMARY

As we advance into an era of serving elders with multiple severe chronic illnesses, we have to strengthen a workforce in the community that can deliver care in the patient's home. Linking many community and medical services with a mobile primary care team that can share in cost savings is our challenge and opportunity. Expansion of PACE, hospice, and IAH models is the future for community-based care of persons with severe chronic illness. We owe this to our elders and to the financial well-being of our society.

REFERENCES

1. Wennberg JE, Fisher ES, Goodman DC, et al. Tracking the care of patients with severe chronic illness. The Dartmouth Atlas of Health Care 2008. Executive Summary April 2008. Available at: www.dartmouthatlas.org. Accessed November 15, 2008.
2. Holtz-Eakin D. High-cost Medicare beneficiaries. Congressional Budget Office. May, 2005. p. 1–12. Available at: http://www.cbo.gov/ftpdocs/63xx/doc6332/05-03-MediSpending.pdf. Accessed October 26, 2008.
3. Guralnick JM, Alecxih L, Branch LG, et al. Medical and long-term care costs when older persons become more dependent. Am J Public Health 2002;92(8):1244–5.
4. Rothman AA, Wagner EH. Chronic illness management: what is the role of primary care? Ann Intern Med 2003;138:256–61.
5. Cigolle CT, Langa KM, Kabeto MU, et al. Setting eligibility criteria for a care-coordination benefit. J Am Geriatr Soc 2005;53(12):2051–9.
6. Orszag P. CBO paper. The Long-Term Budget Outlook. Dec. 2007. p. 19–31. Available at: http://www.cbo.gov/doc.cfm?index=8877. Accessed November 15, 2008.
7. Leff B, Burton L, Mader S, et al. Satisfaction with hospital at home care. J Am Geriatr Soc 2006;54(9):1355–63.
8. Wooldridge J, Brown R, Foster L, et al. Social Health Maintenance Organizations: transition in Medicare + choice. Princeton, NJ: Mathematica Policy Research, Inc.; 2001 [report].
9. Mukamel DB, Peterson DR, Temkin-Greener H, et al. Program characteristics and enrollees' outcomes in the Program of All-Inclusive Care for the Elderly (PACE). Milbank Q 2007;85(3):499–531.
10. Gross DL, Temkin-Greener H, Kunitz S, et al. The growing pains of integrated health care for the elderly: lessons from the expansion of PACE. Milbank Q 2004;82(2):257–82.
11. Temkin-Greener H, Bajorska A, Mukamel DB. Variations in service use in the Program of All-inclusive Care for the Elderly (PACE): is more better? J Gerontol 2008;63(7):731–8.
12. Mukamel DB, Temkin-Greener H, Delavan R, et al. Team performance and risk-adjusted health outcomes in the Program of All-inclusive Care for the Elderly (PACE). Gerontologist 2006;46(2):227–37.

13. Mukamel DB, Peterson DR, Bajorska A, et al. Variations in risk-adjusted outcomes in managed acute/long term care program for frail elderly individuals. Int J for Qual Health Care 2004;16(4):293–301.

14. Grabowski DC. The cost-effectiveness of non-institutional long-term care services: review and synthesis of the most recent evidence. Med Care Res Rev 2006;63(1):3–28.

15. Epping-Jordan JE, Pruitt SD, Bengoa R, et al. Improving the quality of health care for chronic conditions. Qual Saf Health Care 2004;13:299–305.

16. Von Korff M, Gruman JU, Schaefffer J, et al. Collaborative management of chronic illness. Ann Intern Med 1997;127(12):1097–102.

17. Bodenheimer T, Wagner EH, Grumbach K. Improving primary care for patients with chronic illness, part 1. JAMA 2002;288(14):1775–9.

18. Wagner EH, Austin BT, Von Korff M. Organizing care for patients with chronic illness. Milbank Q 1996;74(4):511–44.

19. Coleman K, Mattke S, Perrault PJ, et al. Untangling practice redesign from disease management: how do we best care for the chronically ill? Annu Rev Public Health 2008;30:1.1–1.24.

20. Robert Wood Johnson report. Improving chronic illness care. The Chronic Care Model. Available at: www.improvingchroniccare.org/downloads/rwjf. Accessed November 15, 2008.

21. Bodenheimer T, Wagner EH, Grumbach K. Improving primary care for patients with chronic illness: the chronic care model, part 2. JAMA 2002;288(15):1909–14.

22. Boyd CM, Darer J, Boult C, et al. Clinical practice guidelines and quality of care for older patients with multiple comorbid diseases: implications for pay for performance. JAMA 2005;294(6):716–24.

23. Kemper P. The evaluation of the National Long Term Care Demonstration (10): overview of the findings. Health Serv Res 1988;23(1):161–74.

24. Medicare Health Support Demonstration Program. Center for Medicare and Medicaid. Available at: http://www.cms.hhs.gov/CCIP/downloads/Overview_ketchum_71006.pdf. Accessed November 15, 2008.

25. Abelson R. Medicare finds out how hard it is to save money. NY Times. Available at: http://www.nytimes.com/2008/04/07/business/07medicare.html?_r=1&scp=1&sq=medicare+health+support&st=nyt&oref=slogin. Accessed April 9, 2008.

26. Crippen DL. Disease management in Medicare: data analysis and benefit design issues. Congressional Budget Office September 19, 2002. Available at: http://www.cbo.gov/ftpdocs/37xx/doc3776/09-19-Medicare.pdf. Accessed October 27, 2008.

27. Linden A, Adler-Milstein J. Medicare disease management in policy context. Health Care Financ Rev 2008;29(3):1–11.

28. Chen A, Brown R, Esposito D, et al. Report to Congress on Evaluation of Medicare Disease Management Programs. Princeton, NJ: Mathematica Policy Research; February 2008. PR08-31:47–50.

29. The Advanced Medical Home: A Patient-centered, Physician-guided Model of Health Care. Philadelphia: Policy Monograph of the American College of Physicians; January 16, 2006.

30. Medicare Medical Home Demonstration Project. October 2008. Available at: http://www.cms.hhs.gov/DemoProjectsEvalRpts/downloads/MedHome_FactSheet.pdf. Accessed November 15, 2008.

31. Aging in the United States- Past, Present and Future. Dept. Of Commerce Report. 1997. Available at: http://www.census.gov/ipc/prod/97agewc.pdf. Accessed November 15, 2008.

32. Temkin-Greener H, Bajorska A, Peterson DR, et al. Social support and risk-adjusted mortality in a frail older population. Med Care 2004;42(8):779–88.
33. GAO report the nation's long-term fiscal outlook. August 2007. Available at: http://www.gao.gov/new.items/d071261r.pdf. Accessed November 15, 2008.
34. Paulson HM, Chao EL, Leavitt MO, et al. Status of the social security and Medicare Programs. Summary of 2008 Annual Reports. Available at: http://www.ssa.gov/OACT/TRSUM/trsummary.html. Accessed November 15, 2008.
35. Orszag PR. The Long-term budget outlook and options for slowing the growth of health care costs. Congressional Budget Office, June 17, 2008. Available at: http://www.cbo.gov/ftpdocs/93xx/doc9385/06-17-LTBO_Testimony.pdf. Accessed October 27, 2008.
36. Salsber E, Grover A. Physician workforce shortages: implications and issues for academic health centers and policymakers. Acad Med 2006;81(9):782–7.
37. Goodman DC, Fisher ES. Physician workforce crisis? Wrong diagnosis, wrong prescription. N Engl J Med 2008;358:1658–61.
38. Counsell SR, Callahan CM, Clark DO, et al. Geriatric care management for low-income seniors: a randomized controlled trial. JAMA 2007;298(22):2623–33.
39. Friedrich MJ. Programs bring care to homebound seniors. JAMA 2008;299(22):2618–9.
40. Wachter RM. The state of hospital medicine in 2008. Med Clin North Am 2008;92(2):265–73.

Index

Clin Geriatr Med 25 (2009) 171–177
doi:10.1016/S0749-0690(09)00015-9
geriatric.theclinics.com
0749-0690/09/$ – see front matter © 2009 Elsevier Inc. All rights reserved.

Moving?

Make sure your subscription moves with you!

To notify us of your new address, find your **Clinics Account Number** (located on your mailing label above your name), and contact customer service at:

E-mail: elspcs@elsevier.com

800-654-2452 (subscribers in the U.S. & Canada)
314-453-7041 (subscribers outside of the U.S. & Canada)

Fax number: 314-523-5170

Elsevier Periodicals Customer Service
11830 Westline Industrial Drive
St. Louis, MO 63146

*To ensure uninterrupted delivery of your subscription, please notify us at least 4 weeks in advance of move.

ELSEVIER